Cardiovascular Risk Associated with Schizophrenia and its Treatment

Edited by Professor John Camm

Professor of Clinical Cardiology
Chair of Cardiac and Vascular Department
St.George's Hospital and Medical School
London, UK

First Published 2003 by Galliard Healthcare Communications

© Galliard Healthcare Communications
Fourth Floor, Lincoln House, 296 / 302 High Holborn, London WC1V 7JH
Tel: +44 (0)20 7663 2250
Fax: +44 (0)20 7663 2251

British Library Cataloguing in Publication Data.
A catalogue record for this book is available from the British Library.

ISBN 0-9544351-0-9

Sponsored by an educational grant from Pfizer.

Contents

"Cardiovascular risk associated with schizophrenia and its treatment"

There is an increased mortality seen in people with schizophrenia and sudden death is common. Although some is due to suicide, much is related to significant underlying heart disease. The overall risk of cardiovascular disease, particularly coronary atherosclerosis, is very high in people with schizophrenia and the risk stems from smoking, limited access to medical care, poor judgement about health status, and from the very high prevalence of risk factors amongst this population; diabetes, hypertension, hyperlipidaemia, obesity and metabolic syndrome are all prevalent. Coronary artery disease is therefore more common than in the general adult population.

Some of the sudden death in schizophrenia has been ascribed to therapy with antipsychotic drugs. Some of these drugs have been shown to cause:

- Diabetes and insulin resistance
- Hypercholesterolaemia
- Hypertriglyceridaemia
- Obesity and metabolic syndrome
- Sinus node dysfunction
- α-blockade and neurocardiogenic syncope
- Cardiomyopathy and myocarditis, and
- QT interval prolongation and *torsades de pointes*.

Recent concern has emphasised the potential of antipsychotic drugs to cause ventricular arrhythmias, such as *torsades de pointes*, due to blockade of myocyte membrane currents, prolongation of ventricular repolarisation, QT prolongation on the electrocardiogram, and a re-entrant arrhythmia mechanism. The concern has stemmed from experience with arrhythmias due to "antiarrhythmic" drug treatment, from ventricular arrhythmias due to other medications such as cisapride and terfenadine, and from some experience with antipsychotic medication.

Since sudden death is common in schizophrenia it has been postulated that some deaths may be due to the antipsychotic therapy. Drugs such as thioridazine, pimozide and chlorpromazine, noticeably prolong the QT interval and have been seen to be associated with *torsades de pointes*. Many other antipsychotic medications also prolong the QT interval, but have rarely, if ever, been associated with *torsades de pointes*. By their nature the atypical antipsychotics are relatively new compounds, some of which have only recently been introduced, or are yet to be approved. Consequently, there is not a great deal of experience with their use on which to base confident advice about their potential to induce arrhythmia. However, the risk seems relatively small for many of these agents.

The overall increase in cardiac risk of schizophrenia and its treatment is much more often due to the increased propensity for coronary artery disease. The general risk of *torsades de pointes* is relatively small, but potentially avoidable. In this short book an attempt is made to put into proper perspective the various risk factors for sudden death in schizophrenia.

A. John Camm
Professor of Clinical Cardiology
Chair of Cardiac and Vascular Department
St. George's Hospital and Medical School
London, United Kingdom.

Mortality and sudden death in schizophrenia

Thomas R.E. Barnes[1] and Robert Kerwin[2]

[1]Department of Psychological Medicine, Imperial College, London and

[2]Division of Psychological Medicine, Institute of Psychiatry at the Maudsley, London, United Kingdom

Correspondence: Thomas R.E. Barnes, Professor of Clinical Psychiatry,
Imperial College, Charing Cross Campus, St. Dunstan's Road,
London W6 8RP

1. Mortality in schizophrenia

An increase in mortality in people with psychiatric disorders has been recognised since the 19th century.[1-2] Reviews of mortality studies have concluded that standardised mortality ratios (SMRs) for psychiatric patients, derived from comparisons with the general population and matched control groups, have consistently shown excess mortality from both natural and unnatural causes.[3] More specifically, people with schizophrenia have a substantially increased mortality risk, about twice that of the general population.[4-9] In other words, a proportion of people with schizophrenia will die sooner than would have been expected based on their population birth cohorts.

The first population-based, cause-specific mortality study related to different mental disorders was conducted in Finland.[8] Baseline data were collected between 1977 and 1980 on 8,000 people (4,363 women and 3,637 men) over 30 years of age. For those with schizophrenia, follow-up over 17 years revealed an increased relative risk of death of 3.9 in men and 2.3 in women. The investigators found that the excess mortality was accounted for by cardiovascular disease, respiratory disease, cancer, and, in men, suicide.

In the UK, a 13-year follow-up study was conducted on 370 patients with schizophrenia, who had been ill for an average of 12 years, and most of whom were already middle-aged.[10] The SMRs for all causes (298), and for natural (232) and unnatural causes (1,273), were significantly higher than those to be expected in the general population, as were the SMRs for disease of the circulatory, digestive, endocrine, nervous, and respiratory systems, suicide and undetermined death. The investigators attributed much of this excess mortality to high rates of smoking and unhealthy life style.

2. Natural causes

The reasons for excess mortality in schizophrenia have generally been considered in terms of natural and unnatural causes (see Table 1).[5,11] This is a somewhat uncertain distinction, in that the natural causes listed in Table 1 are not necessarily entirely independent of, and the unnatural causes are not necessarily the direct consequences of, the illness and its treatment. However, the categories provide a convenient basis here for considering causes of premature death in schizophrenia.

Addressing first the natural causes, there are a range of physical illnesses, cardiovascular, respiratory, gastrointestinal, genito-urinary and infective, which are over-represented in people with schizophrenia.[12-15] Underlying the increased risk of such illnesses in people with schizophrenia is a range of unhealthy life style factors, such as heavy smoking, poor nutrition, and a lack of physical exercise.[1,16-18] People with schizophrenia experience a lack of adequate medical and social care, partly because they are less likely to seek and receive appropriate care for medical problems. Phelan and colleagues,[19] suggested that some symptoms of the illness, such as cognitive impairment, social isolation, and suspiciousness, may contribute to individuals not seeking care or adhering to treatment, and their lack of social skills and the stigma of mental illness may compromise the quality of care they receive. Moreover, there is evidence that psychiatrists and general practitioners are poor at recognising and treating physical problems arising in people with severe mental illness.[14,20-22] Generally, the monitoring of physical health and health education in the community in the UK has been considered unsatisfactory (NHS Executive 1999).

Jeste and colleagues,[14] observed that patients with comorbid medical conditions are commonly excluded from research studies, even though they probably represent the majority of individuals with schizophrenia. In addition, smoking-related diseases are more common in people with schizophrenia than in the general population.[10] Indeed, tobacco smoking seems to be particularly associated with schizophrenia compared with other forms of severe mental illness, a relationship that does not seem to be explained in

Table 1. Causes of increased mortality in people with schizophrenia

Natural causes	Unnatural causes
Catatonia	Suicide
	Accidents
Physical illness	Poisoning
Cardiovascular	Violence
Respiratory	
Gastrointestinal	Substance use
Infective	Alcohol
Urogenital	Nicotine
	Illicit drugs (e.g. cannabis, stimulants, opioids)
	Iatrogenic (related to medication)
	Epileptic seizures
	Neuroleptic malignant syndrome
	Agranulocytosis
	Cardiac arrest (e.g. *torsades de pointes*)
	Myocarditis
	Aspiration/asphyxia (choking)
	Respiratory arrest
	Hyperpyrexia
	Circulatory collapse
	Hypothermia
	Sudden unexpected death

(Table 1 adapted from Ref 11. Bandelow B, Fritze J, Rüther E. Increased mortality in schizophrenia and the possible influence of antipsychotic treatment. International Journal of Psychiatry in Clinical Practice (www.tandf.no/ijpcp) 1998; 2 [Suppl 2]: 49–57.)

terms of a link with substance use or institutionalism, or socioeconomic class.[23] The reasons for heavy smoking by people with schizophrenia may relate to a therapeutic effect of nicotine on psychotic symptoms, or an increase in the metabolism of antipsychotic drugs with smoking, leading to a reduction in their side-effects.[14] Brown and colleagues,[10] considered that most of the excess natural mortality of people with schizophrenia in the community was related to cigarette smoking, and that helping patients to stop smoking should be a clinical priority. However, it seems that smoking is not an issue that psychiatrists commonly discuss with their patients with schizophrenia,[24] despite the evidence that simple treatment interventions, such as group work on smoking cessation, can be helpful.[25]

Comorbid substance use is common in people with schizophrenia, particularly alcohol and cannabis, and this has been suggested as a contributory factor to the increased rates of mortality and sudden unexpected death.[26-27] However, in a case control study of medical morbidity, Dalmau and colleagues[28] compared the number of hospitalisations due to somatic disease for 775 people with schizophrenia and controls. They found that the higher incidence of illness in people with schizophrenia was apparent even after exclusion of those who had ever received a diagnosis of substance abuse.

2.1 Cardiovascular causes of death

Cardiovascular mortality of patients with chronic schizophrenia exceeds that of the general population.[12-13] For example, Hannerz and colleagues,[7] showed a significant reduction in life-span of about 10 years in schizophrenia, in part due to increased cardiovascular morbidity. Ösby and colleagues,[29] analysed data from a patient register in Stockholm County, Sweden, and found a doubling of mortality from cardiovascular disease. This increase in cardiovascular-related mortality in schizophrenia may be attributed, at least partly, to the high rates of smoking, obesity, poor diet, and lack of exercise already mentioned, and the relative neglect of these issues in patients with schizophrenia by healthcare professionals.[30] However, the effects of antipsychotic drugs may also contribute to the increase in cardiovascular-related mortality.

Ray and colleagues,[9] conducted a major cohort study of mortality in people receiving antipsychotic drug treatment in the USA. The cohort included 481,744 people, aged 15 to 84 years, enrolled between 1988 and 1993 in Tennessee. On the basis of their daily dosage of antipsychotic medication, each person was categorised as either moderate use (>100mg thioridazine equivalents), low use (<100mg thioridazine equivalents), or non-use. The investigators found that the risk of sudden cardiac death increased with age. Almost half (46%) of the cohort received moderate dosage of conventional antipsychotics. In an analysis of the data that controlled for the effects of smoking, those receiving moderate dosage showed a 2.4 fold increase in the rate of sudden cardiac death compared to those with non-use.

3. Unnatural causes

Simpson and Tsuang (1996)[5] observed that the excess mortality in people with major psychiatric disorder had been attributed to natural causes of death, particularly tuberculosis, pneumonia, infectious diseases and cardiovascular disease. However, the data from their 40-year follow up of a cohort of patients with either schizophrenia or 'atypical' schizophrenia are in accord with those of other studies,[31-32] which suggest that mortality from unnatural causes, particularly suicide, was also excessive over this historical period. Over time, there has been a reduction in mortality related to such natural causes. Thus, consideration of causes of mortality has increasingly focused on unnatural causes, and the possible impact of antipsychotic medication.

For the purpose of examining the role of medication, two studies have compared mortality in psychiatric inpatient populations before and after the introduction of psychotropic drugs.[33-34] No evidence for an increase in overall mortality emerged, although the findings from studies of such a design could be confounded by cohort effects, such as improved nutrition, social conditions and medical and psychiatric care in the later period. More recently, Hiroeh and colleagues[35] carried out one of the largest studies of deaths by unnatural causes. Using the Danish case register they found that 25% of all deaths in psychiatric patients were from unnatural causes, principally homicide, suicide and accident, with SMRs ranging from 300 – 1300.

3.1 Weight gain and diabetes

An increase in body weight with conventional antipsychotic drugs, particularly the so-called low-potency drugs such as chlorpromazine, has been recognised for decades. For example, obesity of a clinically-significant degree has been reported in about a third of patients receiving maintenance treatment with depot injections of fluphenazine decanoate or flupenthixol decanoate, which represents an increase in the prevalence of about four times compared with that in the general population.[36] This has implications for the general health of the patients prescribed such medication, as obesity is a powerful, independent risk factor for serious medical conditions such as type II diabetes, hypertension, coronary heart disease, and osteoarthritis.[36-37] Weight gain can also be stigmatising, and contribute to poor compliance.

The newer, atypical antipsychotics are now widely used, and their main advantage is a lower liability for extrapyramidal side-effects such as parkinsonism, akathisia and acute dystonia, and there is also preliminary evidence for a lower risk of tardive dyskinesia with some of these drugs.[38] However, they are also associated with a range of side-effects that overlap with those of the conventional drugs, and these include weight gain, disturbance of glucose metabolism, and increased concentrations of blood cholesterol and lipids. All atypical antipsychotics may potentially cause weight gain, but there is a marked variability among the atypical agents in their tendency to promote an increase in body weight.[39–40] The drugs most commonly implicated are clozapine[37,41–42] and olanzapine.[43–44] Possible predictors of increased weight include age, baseline body mass index, appetite stimulation, previous antipsychotic exposure, and duration of antipsychotic treatment.[45] An association between antipsychotic-induced weight gain and therapeutic response to medication has been suggested, with those patients likely to have the greatest antipsychotic benefit from olanzapine or clozapine treatment being at the highest risk of a clinically significant increase in weight gain.[46]

In addition, a relatively high prevalence of type II diabetes mellitus and impaired glucose tolerance in people with schizophrenia receiving antipsychotic medication has been reported.[47] Impaired glucose metabolism was first reported in people with psychotic illness before the introduction of antipsychotic medication. However, treatment with such medication is associated with impaired glucose metabolism, exacerbation of existing diabetes, new-onset type II diabetes mellitus, as well as diabetic ketoacidosis,[48] although the mechanism remains uncertain. Antipsychotics can increase abdominal adiposity, and this can decrease insulin sensitivity, which may explain some of the changes seen in glucose metabolism. However, adverse effects on glucose metabolism may be occurring with some antipsychotics independent of adiposity.[49–50] The comorbid presence of diabetes with schizophrenia may contribute to the raised mortality of such patients.[4,49,51–52] Type II diabetes is associated with an increased risk of hypertension and coronary artery disease, and Haupt and Newcomer (2001)[49] noted that a relationship between plasma glucose levels and cardiovascular risk, such as myocardial infarction or stroke, may develop at glucose levels that are significantly below the recognised diabetic thresholds. Atypical antipsychotics may be more likely to cause diabetes than conventional drugs. For example, a data-mining study by Sernyak and colleagues,[53] examined database information on 38,632 outpatients with schizophrenia treated with conventional and atypical antipsychotics in the USA over a four-month period in 1999. Controlling for the effects of age, those individuals receiving atypical drugs were 9% more likely to have diabetes than those on conventional drugs. It is possible that the individual atypical drugs differ in their propensity to cause diabetes, but the findings of studies so far do not allow for any confident statements about relative liability.[54]

The lack of definitive recommendations reveals the need for detailed clinical and health economic research on patients receiving various antipsychotic drugs, examining cardiovascular risk profiles in terms of weight gain, risk of diabetes and lipid changes (e.g. hypercholesterolaemia and hypertriglyceridaemia).

3.2 Sudden unexpected death

Sudden, unexpected, unexplained death can be defined[55] as death within one hour of symptoms (excluding suicide, homicide and accident)[56] which is both unexpected in relation to the degree of disability before death,[57] and unexplained because clinical investigation and autopsy failed to identify any plausible cause.[58] There have been numerous reports of such deaths in people with mental health problems taking antipsychotic medication.[26,59] Some of these cases have involved high doses of antipsychotics, polypharmacy, and the use of drugs no longer commonly used in clinical practice. Nevertheless, the possible association between antipsychotic drugs and sudden death has been a source of professional and public concern for several decades.[60]

Estimating the frequency of sudden death is rather uncertain. Ray and colleagues,[9] suggested that sudden unexpected death occurs twice as often in individuals receiving antipsychotic medication than in the normal population, but Glassman and Bigger (2001)[61] determined that it remains a rare event, with only 10 to 15 such events occurring in 50,000 person-years of observation, although the rate will be strongly influenced by age, gender and particularly the presence of cardiac disease. Glassman and Bigger

(2001)[61] calculated that over a 10-year period of exposure to antipsychotic drugs there would be four additional deaths in 1,000 medically healthy young or middle-aged patients receiving antipsychotic medication compared with matched subjects, and that only one or two of these deaths might be accounted for by differences between antipsychotics.

3.2.1 Cardiac causes

Antipsychotic drugs have effects on cardiac function, particularly prolongation of the QT interval, the clinical significance of which remains unclear. However, one possible mechanism for sudden unexpected death is that prolonged QTc (QT interval corrected for heart rate), reflecting abnormal cardiac repolarisation, may increase the risk of developing potentially serious ventricular arrhythmias, such as *torsades de pointes*. Algra and colleagues,[62] found that QTc prolongation was an independent risk factor for sudden death in individuals without intra-ventricular conduction defects.

Glassman and Bigger (2001)[61] reviewed the risks of prolonged QT interval, *torsades de pointes* and sudden death with antipsychotic drugs. They concluded that while pimozide, sertindole, droperidol and haloperidol had all been documented to cause *torsades de pointes* and sudden death, the greatest risk was with thioridazine. Thioridazine was one of the most widely prescribed antipsychotic drugs in the UK, being particularly commonly used in the elderly. It was implicated in a Finnish study of sudden death in patients on normal doses of psychotropic drugs.[63] Mehtonen and colleagues,[63] examined all coroner's cases in Finland over three years (1985–1988). Of the 24,000 records studied, there were 49 sudden unexpected deaths in apparently healthy adults receiving psychotropic medication, and the data suggested an association with low-potency phenothiazine antipsychotics, particularly thioridazine. In the UK, in February 2001, the Committee on Safety of Medicines (CSM) had received 42 UK reports of suspected heart rate and rhythm disorders since 1964.[64] Out of the 39 cases where the outcome was known, 21 were reported as fatal.[64] In December 2000, the risk:benefit balance ratio was considered to be favourable only as second line treatment for schizophrenia. The CSM further recommended that thioridazine was not to be used for sedation or to treat agitation in the elderly, and the advice included ECG screening and monitoring, specifically that, all patients should have baseline ECG screening and electrolytes measured. These should be repeated at each dose escalation and at six monthly intervals.

Reilly and colleagues,[65] have reported an increased risk of QT interval prolongation for both thioridazine and droperidol. Droperidol showed lengthening of cardiac repolarisation and dose-dependent increases in QTc interval.[66–67] From 1993–1999 the manufacturers of droperidol received 72 cases of QT prolongation, serious ventricular arrhythmia or sudden death worldwide. The drug was voluntarily discontinued in 2001.[64]

Several more recent antipsychotic drugs have been implicated in cases of sudden unexpected death. Pimozide was associated with 13 unexpected deaths. Ten of the individuals had been receiving more than 20 mg per day, and seven were under 30 years of age. Most had no previously known cardiac abnormality, and most had received a rapid increase in dose. Dose restrictions were subsequently recommended (lowering the upper dose from 60 to 20 mg per day) and ECG monitoring advised.[68] However, a Cochrane systematic review of 34 randomised studies failed to find evidence of higher mortality with pimozide.[69]

In December 1998, the manufacturers of the atypical antipsychotic sertindole voluntarily suspended the drug due to concerns about cardiac arrhythmia and sudden cardiac death associated with its use.[70–71] Subsequently, the issue was re-evaluated within the European licensing procedures, and new pre-clinical and epidemiological data were considered. In 2002, a restricted reintroduction of sertindole was approved, with a number of safeguards. Initially, it was only to be given to patients enrolled in clinical studies.

A definite causal link between drug treatment and sudden death has yet to be demonstrated. Most studies of sudden unexpected death have been retrospective with no comparison group, and follow-up studies have generally suggested that the incidence is low.[72–73] Following a comprehensive review of the literature, Simpson and colleagues[59] concluded: "Although a relationship between the use of antipsychotic drugs and sudden death has not been firmly established, it has also not been disproved." A review 10 years later[26] came to a similar conclusion: "There are insufficient epidemiological data to prove that sudden death is more likely amongst people being treated with antipsychotic medication than it is amongst the general population. However, there are no data that prove there is no causal relationship between the use of this group of drugs and sudden death." Nevertheless, high dose and increasing age have been identified as risk factors for QTc prolongation,[65,74] and exposure to thioridazine, droperidol and tricyclic antidepressants emerged as independent risk factors in the study of Reilly and colleagues,[65] with thioridazine being the strongest risk factor.

Myocarditis presents with fever, chest pain, dyspnoea, tachycardia and fatigue, and can be fatal. The atypical antipsychotic, clozapine, has been reported to cause both myocarditis and cardiomyopathy.[75-77] Kilian and colleagues,[76] reported on 8,000 patients started on clozapine treatment in Australia between 1990 and 1997. In total, there were five cases of myocarditis (five fatal) and eight who developed cardiomyopathy (one fatal). The median exposure to clozapine was 15 days. The investigators calculated the fatal myocarditis risk as 1 in 500, although this may be higher than in other countries.[78] Suggested pathophysiological mechanisms include genetic predisposition, interaction of drug-environmental factors, and association with metabolic side-effects.[79-80] Warner and colleagues,[78] questioned these findings on the basis that myocarditis symptoms might overlap with drug effects, and that individuals with treatment-resistant schizophrenia may be at increased risk of such problems.

Coulter and colleagues,[81] conducted a data mining study, examining a World Health Organisation (WHO) international database on adverse drug reactions. They found that cardiomyopathy and myocarditis were significantly more frequently reported with clozapine. However, there were also associations between myocarditis or cardiomyopathy and other atypical antipsychotics (risperidone), some conventional antipsychotics (chlorpromazine, fluphenazine and haloperidol), and lithium, which these investigators considered warranted further study.

3.2.2 Non-cardiac causes

In 1987, reports by The Royal College of Psychiatrists[26] and Simpson and colleagues,[59] considered the occurrence of sudden unexpected death in the general population and the non-drug causes that could account for deaths in those with psychiatric illness. For example, a syndrome of sudden death in psychiatric patients, variously called acute exhaustive mania or lethal catatonia, among other names, was noted prior to the introduction of antipsychotic medication.[82-83] This condition was characterised by persistent and extreme psychomotor excitement, leading to unexpected collapse and death, although it would not be accurate to refer to this as an unexplained death.

Psychological stress and strenuous exercise have been identified as factors related to sudden death in the general population,[84] and both may be relevant in some cases of sudden death in people with psychotic illness, for example when they are being restrained.[85] A possible mechanism is a marked increase in circulating levels of the catecholamines, noradrenaline and adrenaline, and excess vagal and adrenergic stimulation. Such sympathetic over-stimulation and adrenaline release may increase myocardial excitability, and lead to fatal cardiac arrhythmia. This notion is compatible with the reports of fatal collapse of athletes during the height of physical activity or young soldiers during physically-demanding exercises,[86-87] and the finding that animals placed in restraint have an increased frequency of cardiac arrhythmias, and some will die in this situation.[88] Other, non-cardiac causes of sudden unexpected death include convulsions, hyperpyrexia, vasodilatation and hypotension, and aspiration and asphyxia related to factors such as an impaired gag reflex and laryngeal-pharyngeal dystonia.[26,59,89]

4. Suicide

Patients with schizophrenia seem to be at greater risk of dying from self-neglect and malnutrition, suicide, accidents and murder.[32,35,90-91] Suicide remains the commonest cause,[51,92] with estimates of the completed suicide rate for individuals with schizophrenia at about 10%.[92-93] Reported SMRs for schizophrenia in the literature have varied between 6,000 at worst and 1,666 at best.[94] Large follow-up studies of mortality in first-admission patients with schizophrenia conducted in Sweden and Denmark[12,95] revealed high SMRs for suicide. Both groups of investigators commented on the relatively high proportion of deaths by suicide in younger patients, particularly in males, during the early stages of the illness following first admission. Mortensen and Juel (1993)[12] speculated that an increasing suicide risk over recent years in some countries might partly reflect the adverse effects of deinstitutionalisation, a point echoed by Stephens and colleagues.[96]

The frequency of suicide attempts in people with schizophrenia is higher than that for completed suicide. For example, a survey of individuals with schizophrenia and bipolar disorder reported that 19% had threatened or attempted suicide within the previous year[97], and the Epidemiologic Catchment Area study in the USA reported that 28% of people with schizophrenia had attempted suicide.[98] Risk factors for suicide attempts include the presence of positive psychotic symptoms at the time[99] and, perhaps more specifically, suspiciousness and delusions, which Fenton and colleagues[100] found to be more severe among successful suicides. Inadequate maintenance of care and treatment, including poor adherence to drug treatment regimens, may also be risk factors for suicide.[101–102]

Weighing up the risks and benefits of antipsychotic medication should take account of emerging evidence of some advantages for clozapine, and possibly other atypical antipsychotics, in reducing suicide in schizophrenia and schizoaffective disorder.[103] Meltzer and Okayli (1995)[104] were the first to observe about an 80% reduction in suicidal ideation in their patients being treated with clozapine. This effect was also observed in a large, epidemiological cohort of over 67,000 clozapine-treated patients in the USA, in which the suicide rate was reduced to 0.18 of the expected rate.[105] This latter study also found reduced rates of both natural and unnatural causes of death with clozapine. Munro and colleagues,[94] confirmed this finding in a UK cohort of 12,760, where the SMR for suicide was reduced to 498. An international suicide prevention trial comparing clozapine with olanzapine in suicidal patients, demonstrated probable overall reduced rates of suicide for both drugs compared with historical controls and superiority for clozapine in preventing suicide attempts.[106] Modeling the data from Walker and colleagues[105] and Munro and colleagues[94] to calculate lives potentially saved from suicide, shows that between 200 – 500 lives in the UK may be saved over a 10-year period, depending on the specific constraints of the model.[107]

Data concerning the anti-suicidal effect of other antipsychotics is limited. However, there is preliminary evidence that some may have a beneficial effect, although this effect is limited to retrospective analyses in short-term studies in patient populations not unduly at risk.[108–109] Further prospective studies are currently underway.

In summary, how does the possible reduction in suicide rate with some of the newer antipsychotic drugs balance up against the risks of increased mortality and morbidity associated with weight gain and diabetes induced by these agents? Relevant evidence was provided by Fontaine and colleagues,[52] who assessed the impact of antipsychotic-induced weight gain and impaired glucose tolerance in schizophrenia and applied data from the Framingham USA heart study to predict risk. Fontaine and colleagues,[52] calculated that with the use of clozapine there would be 416 additional deaths due to weight gain per 100,000 patients treated, compared with 492 lives that might be expected to be saved from suicide.

References

1. Gausset MF, Casadebaig JM, Guillaud-Bataille N, et al. Mortality among the mentally ill: A review. L' Encéphale 1992; XVIII: 93 – 100 [Abstract].

2. McColl AJ, Gulliford MC. Population health outcome indicators for the NHS: A feasibility study. London: Faculty of Public Health Medicine and the Department of Public Health Medicine, United Medical and Dental schools of Guy's and St Thomas' Hospitals, 1993

3. Harris EC, Barraclough B. Excess mortality of mental disorder. Br Journal Psychiatry 1998; 173: 11–53.

4. Allebeck P. Schizophrenia: A life-shortening disease. Schizophr Bull 1989; 15: 81–89.

5. Simpson JC, Tsuang MT. Mortality among patients with schizophrenia. Schizophr Bull 1996; 22: 485–499.

6. Brown S. Excess mortality of schizophrenia: A meta-analysis. Br J Psychiatry 1997; 171: 502–508.

7. Hannerz H, Bolga P, Borritz M. Life expectancies for individuals with psychiatric diagnoses. Public Health 2001; 115: 328–337.

8. Joukamaa M, Heliovaara M, Knekt P et al. Mental disorders and cause-specific mortality. Br J Psychiatry 2001; 179: 498–502.

9. Ray WA, Meredith S, Thapa PB, et al. Antipsychotics and the risk of sudden cardiac death. Arch Gen Psychiatry 2001; 58: 1161–1167.

10. Brown S, Inskip H, Barraclough B. Causes of the excess mortality of schizophrenia. Br J Psychiatry 2000; 177: 212–217.

11. Bandelow B, Fritze J, Rüther E. Increased mortality in schizophrenia and the possible influence of antipsychotic treatment. Int J Psych Clin Prac 1998; 2 (Suppl 2): 49–57.

12. Mortensen PB, Juel L. Mortality and causes of death in schizophrenic patients in Denmark. Acta Psychiatr Scand 1990; 81: 372–377.

13. Newman SC, Bland RC. Mortality in a cohort of patients with schizophrenia: A record linkage study. Can J Psychiatry 1991; 36: 239–245.

14. Jeste DV, Gladsjo JA, Lindamer LA, et al. Medical comorbidity in schizophrenia. Schizophr Bull 1996; 22: 413–430.

15. Kendrick T. Cardiovascular and respiratory risk factors and symptoms among general practice patients with long-term mental illness. Br J Psychiatry 1996; 169: 733–739.

16. Lesage AD, Trapani V, Tansella M. Excess mortality by natural causes of Italian schizophrenic patients. Eur Arch Psychiatr Neurol Sci 1990; 239: 361–365.

17. Brown S, Birtwhistle J, Roe L, et al. The unhealthy lifestyle of people with schizophrenia. Psychol Med 1999; 29: 697–701.

18. Bralet MC, Yon V, Loas G, et al. Mortality in schizophrenia: A 8-year follow-up study in 150 chronic schizophrenics. L' Encéphale 2000; XXVI: 32–41 [Abstract].

19. Phelan M, Stradins L, Morrison S. Physical health of people with severe mental illness. BMJ 2001; 322: 442–444.

20. Gournay K. Setting clinical standards for care in schizophrenia. Nurs Times 1996; 92: 36–37.

21. Felker B, Yazel JJ, Short D. Mortality and medical comorbidity among psychiatric patients: A review. *Psychiatr Serv* 1996; **47**: 1356–1363.

22. Osborn DPJ. The poor physical health of people with mental illness. *West J Med* 2001; **175**: 329–332.

23. de Leon J, Tracy J, McCann E, *et al*. Schizophrenia and tobacco smoking: A replication study in another US psychiatric hospital. *Schizophr Res* 2002; **56**: 55–65.

24. Lawrie SM, Hutchison JK, Sweeney SR, *et al*. Psychosis and substance abuse: Cause, effect or coincidence? *Scott Med J* 1995; **40**: 174–176.

25. Addington J, el-Guebaly N, Campbell W, *et al*. Smoking cessation treatment for patients with schizophrenia. *Am J Psychiatry* 1998; **155**: 974–976.

26. Report of the working group of the Royal College of Psychiatrists' Psychopharmacology Sub-Group. Council Report CR57. *The association between antipsychotic drugs and sudden death*. London: Royal College of Psychiatrists, 1997; pp15.

27. Ruschena D, Mullen PE, Burgess P, *et al*. Sudden death in psychiatric patients. *Br J Psychiatry* 1998; **172**: 331–336.

28. Dalmau A, Bergman B, Brismar B. Somatic morbidity in schizophrenia – A case control study. *Public Health* 1997; **111**: 393–397.

29. Ösby U, Correia N, Brandt L, *et al*. Time trends in schizophrenia mortality in Stockholm County, Sweden: Cohort study. *BMJ* 2000; **321**: 483–484.

30. Le Fevre PD. Improving the physical health of patients with schizophrenia: Therapeutic nihilism or realism? *Scott Med J* 2001; **46**: 11–13.

31. Temoche A, Pugh TF, MacMahon B. Suicide rates among current and former mental institution patients. *J Nervous Ment Dis* 1964; **138**: 124–130.

32. Tsuang MT, Woolson RF. Excess mortality in schizophrenia and affective disorders.: Do suicides and accidental deaths solely account for this excess? *Arch Gen Psychiatry* 1978; **35**: 1181–1185.

33. Brill H, Patton RE. Clinical statistical analysis of population changes in New York State Mental Hospital since the introduction of psychotropic drugs. *Am J Psychiatry* 1962; **119**: 20–35.

34. Craig TJ, Lin SP. Mortality among psychiatric inpatients: Age-adjusted comparison of populations before and after psychotropic drug era. *Arch Gen Psychiatry* 1981; **38**: 935–938.

35. Hiroeh U, Appleby L, Mortensen PB, *et al*. Death by homicide, suicide, and other unnatural causes in people with mental illness: A population-based study. *Lancet* 2001; **358**: 2110–2112.

36. Silverstone T, Elmslie J. Body weight changes during treatment with psychotropic drugs. *Psychiatrists' Information Service Monograph Series, Number 3*. Cheshire: Gardiner-Caldwell Communications, 1995.

37. Umbricht D, Kane JM. Medical complications of new antipsychotic drugs. *Schizophr Bull* 1996; **22**: 475–483.

38. Barnes TRE, McPhillips MA. Critical analysis and comparison of the side-effect and safety profiles of the new antipsychotics. *Br J Psychiatry* 1999; **174(Suppl 38)**: 34–43.

39. Allison DB, Mentore JL, Heo M, *et al*. Antipsychotic-induced weight gain: A comprehensive research synthesis. *Am J Psychiatry* 1999; **156**: 1686–1696.

40. Simpson MM, Goetz RR, Devlin MJ, *et al*. Weight gain and antipsychotic medication: Differences between antipsychotic-free and treatment periods. *J Clin Psychiatry* 2001; **62**: 694–700.

41. Hummer M, Kemmler G, Kurz M, *et al*. Weight gain induced by clozapine. *Eur Neuropsychopharmacol* 1995; **5**: 437–440.

42. Briffa D, Meehan T. Weight changes during clozapine treatment. *Aust N Z J Psychiatry* 1998; **32**: 718–21.

43. Beasley Jr CM, Tollefson GD, Tran PV. Safety of olanzapine. *J Clin Psychiatry* 1997; **5(Suppl 10)**: 13–17.

44. Duggan L, Fenton M, Dardennes RM, *et al*. Olanzapine for schizophrenia. *The Cochrane Library, Issue 4*. Oxford: Update Software Ltd, 2002.

45. McIntyre RS, McCann SM, Kennedy SH. Antipsychotic metabolic effects: Weight gain, diabetes mellitus, and lipid abnormalities. *Can J Psychiatry* 2001; **46**: 273–281.

46. Czobor P, Volavka J, Sheitman B, *et al*. Antipsychotic-induced weight gain and therapeutic response: A differential association. *J Clin Psychopharmacol* 2002; **22**: 244–251.

47. Brambilla F, Guastalla A, Guerrini A, *et al*. Glucose-insulin metabolism in chronic schizophrenia. *Dis Nerv Syst* 1976; **37**: 98–103.

48. Jin H, Meyer JM, Jeste DV. Phenomenology of and risk factors for new-onset diabetes mellitus and diabetic ketoacidosis associated with atypical antipsychotics: An analysis of 45 published cases. *Ann Clin Psychiatry* 2002; **14**: 59–64.
49. Haupt DW, Newcomer JW. Hyperglycaemia and antipsychotic medications. *J Clin Psychiatry* 2001; **62(Suppl 27)**: 15–26.
50. Newcomer JW, Haupt DW, Fucetola R, *et al.* Abnormalities in glucose regulation during antipsychotic treatment of schizophrenia. *Arch Gen Psychiatry* 2002; **59**: 337–345.
51. Harris EC, Barraclough B. Suicide as an outcome for mental disorders. *Br J Psychiatry* 1997; **170**: 205–208.
52. Fontaine KR, Heo M, Halligan EP, *et al.* Estimating the consequences of anti-psychotic induced weight gain on health and mortality rate. *Psychiatry Res* 2001; **101**: 277–288.
53. Sernyak MJ, Leslie DL, Alarcon RD, *et al.* Association of diabetes mellitus with use of atypical neuroleptics in the treatment of schizophrenia. *Am J Psychiatry* 2002; **159**: 561–566.
54. Koro CE, Fedder DO, L'Italien GJ, *et al.* Assessment of independent effect of olanzapine and risperidone on risk of diabetes among patients with schizophrenia: Population based nested case-control study. *BMJ* 2002; **325**: 243.
55. Jusic N, Lader M. Post-mortem antipsychotic drug concentrations and unexplained deaths. *Br J Psychiatry* 1994; **165**: 787–791.
56. Ungvari G. Neuroleptic-related sudden death: Proven or a mere hypothesis? *Pharmacopsychiatry* 1980; **13**: 29.
57. Kuller L, Lilienfield A, Fisher R. An epidemiological study of sudden and unexpected deaths in adults. *Medicine* 1967; **46**: 341–361.
58. Hirsch CS, Martin DL. Unexpected death in young epileptics. *Neurology* 1971; **21**: 682.
59. Simpson GM, Davis J, Jefferson JW, *et al. Sudden deaths in psychiatric patients: The role of neuroleptic drugs.* Washington DC: American Psychiatric Association Task Force Report No. 27, 1987
60. Appleby L ,Thomas S, Ferrier N, *et al.* Sudden unexplained death in psychiatric in-patients. *Br J Psychiatry* 2000; **176**: 405–406.
61. Glassman AH, Bigger, Jr., JT. Antipsychotic drugs: Prolonged QTc interval, *torsades de pointes*, and sudden death. *Am J Psychiatry* 2001; **158**: 1774–1782.
62. Algra A, Tijssen JGP, Roelandt JRCT, *et al.* QTc prolongation measured by standard 12-lead electrocardiography is an independent risk factor for sudden death due to cardiac arrest. *Circulation* 1991; **83**: 1888–1894.
63. Mehtonen OP, Aranko K, Malkonen L, *et al.* A survey of sudden death associated with the use of antipsychotic or antidepressant drugs: 49 cases in Finland. *Acta Psychiatrica Scandinavica* 1991; **84**: 58–64.
64. Committee on Safety of Medicines and Medicines Control Agency. QT interval prolongation with antipsychotics. *Curr Problems in Pharmacovigilance* 2001; **27**: 4.
65. Reilly JG, Ayis SA, Ferrier IN, *et al.* QTc-interval abnormalities and psychotropic drug therapy in psychiatric patients. *Lancet* 2000; **355**: 1048–1052.
66. Lischke V, Behne M, Doelken P, *et al.* Droperidol causes a dose-dependent prolongation of the QT interval. *Anesth Analg* 1994; **79**: 983–986.
67. Drolet B, Zhang S, Deschenes D, *et al.* Droperidol lengthens cardiac repolarization due to block of the rapid component of the delayed rectifier potassium current. *J Cardiovasc Electrophysiol* 1999; **10**: 1597–1604.
68. Committee on Safety of Medicines. Cardiotoxic effects of Pimozide. *Curr Problems in Pharmacovigilance* 1990; **16**: 29.
69. Sultana A, McGonagle T. Pimozide for schizophrenia or related psychoses. *The Cochrane Library, Issue 4.* Oxford: Update Software Ltd, 2002.
70. Wilton LV, Heeley EL, Pickering RM, *et al.* Comparative study of mortality rates and cardiac dysrhythmias in post-marketing surveillance studies of sertindole and two other atypical drugs, risperidone and olanzapine. *J Psychopharmacol* 2001; **15**: 120–126.
71. Committee on Safety of Medicines. Suspension of Availability of Sertindole (Serdolect). *Curr Problems in Pharmacovigilance* 1999; **25**: 1.
72. Swett CP, Shader RI. Cardiac side-effects and sudden death in hospitalized psychiatric patients. *Dis Nerv Syst* 1977; **38**: 69–72.
73. Goldney RD, Spence ND, Bowes JA. Clinical report: The safe use of high-dose

neuroleptics in a psychiatric intensive care unit. *Aust N Z J Psychiatry* 1986; **20**: 370–375.

74. Warner JP, Barnes TRE, Henry J. Electrocardiographic changes in patients receiving neuroleptic medication. *Acta Psychiatrica Scandinavica* 1996; **93**: 311–313.

75. Jensen VE, Gotzsche O. Allergic myocarditis in clozapine treatment. *Ugeskrift for Laeger* 1994; **156**: 4151–4152 [German].

76. Killian JG, Kerr K, Lawrence C, *et al*. Myocarditis and cardiomyopathy associated with clozapine. *Lancet* 1999; **354**: 1841–1845.

77. La Grenade L, Graham D, Trontell A. Myocarditis and cardiomyopathy associated with clozapine use in the United States. *N Engl J Med* 2001; **345**: 224–225.

78. Warner B, Alphs L, Schaedelin J, *et al*. Clozapine and sudden death. *Lancet* 2000; **355**: 842.

79. Devarajan S, Kutcher SP, Dursun SM. Clozapine and sudden death. *Lancet* 2000; **355**: 841.

80. Chan NN. Clozapine and sudden death. *Lancet* 2000; **355**: 841–842.

81. Coulter DM, Bate A, Meyboom RHB, *et al*. Antipsychotic drugs and heart muscle disorder in international pharmacovigilance: Data mining study. *BMJ* 2001; **322**: 1207–1209.

82. Bell LV. On a form of disease resembling some advanced stages of mania and fever, but so contradistinguished from any ordinarily observed or described combination of symptoms, as to render it probable that it may be an overlooked and hitherto unrecorded malady. *Am J Insanity* 1849; **6**: 97–127.

83. Adland ML. Review, case studies, therapy and interpretation of the acute exhaustive psychoses. *Psychiatr Q* 1947; **21**: 38–69.

84. O'Halloran RL, Lewman LV. Restraint asphyxiation in excited delirium. *Am J Forensic Med Pathol* 1993; **14**: 289–295.

85. Banerjee S, Bingley W, Murphy E. *Deaths of Detained Patients: A Review of Reports to the Mental Health Act Commission*. London: Mental Health foundation, 1995.

86. Phillips M, Robinowitz M, Higgins JR, *et al*. Sudden cardiac death in Air Force recruits. A 20 year review. *JAMA* 1986; **256**: 2696–2699.

87. Hillis WS, McIntyre PD, Maclean J, *et al*. Sudden death in sport. *BMJ* 1994; **309**: 657–660.

88. Dimsdale JE. Emotional causes of sudden death. *Am J Psychiatry* 1977; **134**: 1361–1366.

89. Brown RP, Kocsis JH. Sudden death and antipsychotic drugs. *Hosp Community Psychiatry* 1984; **35**: 486–491.

90. Tsuang MT, Woolson RF, Fleming JA. Causes of death in schizophrenia and manic-depression. *Br J Psychiatry* 1980; **136**: 239–242.

91. Black DW, Fisher R. Mortality in DSM-IIIR schizophrenia. *Schizophr Res* 1992; **7**: 109–116.

92. Caldwell CB, Gottesman II. Schizophrenics kill themselves too: A review of risk factors for suicide. *Schizophr Bull* 1990; **16**: 571–589.

93. Siris SG. Suicide and schizophrenia. *J Psychopharmacol* 2001; **15**: 127–135.

94. Munro J, O'Sullivan D, Andrews C, *et al*. Active monitoring of 12,760 clozapine recipients in the UK and Ireland: Beyond pharmacovigilance. *Br J Psychiatry* 1999; **175**: 576–580.

95. Ösby U, Correia N, Brandt L, *et al*. Mortality and causes of death in schizophrenia in Stockholm County, Sweden. *Schizophr Res* 2000; **45**: 21–28.

96. Stephens J, Richard P, McHugh PR. Suicide in patients hospitalized for schizophrenia: 1913–1940. *J Nerv Ment Dis* 1999; **187**: 10–14.

97. Steinwachs DM *et al*. F*amily perspectives on meeting the needs for care of severely mentally ill relatives: A national survey*. Maryland: School of Public Hygiene and Public Health, Johns Hopkins University, 1992

98. Robins LN, Regier DA. *Psychiatric Disorders in America*. New York: Free Press, 1991; pp50.

99. Nieto E, Vieta E, Gasto C, *et al*. Suicide attempts of high medical seriousness in schizophrenic patients. *Compr Psychiatry* 1992; **33**: 384–387.

100. Fenton WS, McGlashan TH, Victor BJ, *et al*. Symptoms, subtype, and suicidality in patients with schizophrenia spectrum disorders. *Am J Psychiatry* 1997; **154**: 199–204.

101. Appleby L, Shaw J, Amos T, *et al*. Suicide within 12 months of contact with mental health services: National clinical survey. *BMJ* 1999; **318**: 1235–1239.

102. De Hert M, McKenzie K, Peuskens J. Risk factors for suicide in young people suffering from schizophrenia: A long-term follow-up study. *Schizophr Res* 2001; **47**: 127–134.

103. Reid WH, Mason M, Hogan T. Suicide prevention effects associated with clozapine therapy in schizophrenia and schizoaffective disorder. *Psychiatr Serv* 1998; **49**: 1029–1033.

104. Meltzer HY, Okayli G. Reduction of suicidality during clozapine treatment of neuroleptic resistant schizophrenia: Impact on risk benefit assessment. *Am J Psychiatry* 1995; **152**: 183–190.

105. Walker AM, Lanza LL, Arellano F, *et al.* Mortality in current and former users of clozapine. *Epidemiology* 1997; **8**: 671–677.

106. Meltzer HY, Alphs L, Green AI, *et al.* Clozapine treatment for suicidality in schizophrenia: International Suicide Prevention Trial (InterSePT). *Arch Gen Psychiatry* 2003; **60**: 82–91.

107. Warren, Knapp, Kerwin submitted. *British Journal of Psychiatry* 2003 – In Press.

108. Tran PV, Hamilton SH, Kuntz AJ, *et al.* Double blind comparison of olanzapine verses risperidone in the treatment of schizophrenia and other psychotic disorders. *J Clin Psychopharmacol* 1997; **17**: 407–419.

109. Khan A, Khan SR, Leventhal RM, *et al.* Symptom reduction and suicide risk among patients treated with placebo in antipsychotic clinical trials: an analysis of the food and drug administration database. *Am J Psychiatry* 2001; **158**: 1449–1454.

Adverse metabolic effects of atypical antipsychotics

[1]Ali Dana and [2]Michael Marber

[1]Specialist Registrar in Cardiology, St Thomas' Hospital, London

[2]Professor of Cardiology and Honorary Consultant Cardiologist

Guy's, King's & St Thomas' Medical School, London, United Kingdom

Correspondence: Professor Michael Marber, Department of Cardiology, King's College London, The Rayne Institute, St Thomas' Hospital, London SE1 7EH

1. Introduction

Mortality from coronary heart disease has declined steadily in industrialised countries in the past 20 to 30 years due to primary and secondary prevention, and to improved treatment of its acute manifestations.[1-2] Unfortunately, however, coronary disease remains the leading cause of death in the developed world. The evidence that most cardiovascular disease is preventable continues to grow, and results of long-term prospective studies consistently identify persons with low levels of defined risk factors as having a low lifelong risk of heart disease and stroke.[3] These findings have focused attention on primary prevention of cardiovascular disease in prospectively identified high-risk individuals. In the late 1990's, guidelines were published by American and European task forces, outlining simple recommendations on detection and management of established risk factors for coronary disease.[4-5] In all of these guidelines, there is an increasing emphasis on stratifying patients by level of risk and matching the intensity of interventions to the hazard for cardiovascular disease events. For instance, in the European guidelines, the stated priorities lay with secondary and 'high risk' primary prevention when the estimated risk of a coronary heart disease event over 10 years is greater than 20%.[5]

The more established risk factors for coronary atherosclerosis are outlined in Table 1. These can be either modifiable or non-modifiable. Non-modifiable risk factors include the male gender, advancing age, and a family history of

Table 1. Risk factors for coronary heart disease.

Modifiable	Non-modifiable
Diabetes mellitus	Gender
Hypertension	Age
Smoking	Family History
Physical inactivity	
Hypercholesterolaemia	
Obesity	
Hypertriglyceridaemia	
No daily alcohol intake	

(Adapted from Ref 32. Kurzthaler I, Fleischehacker WW. The clinical implications of weight gain in schizophrenia. *J Clin Psychiatry* 62 [Suppl 7]: 32–37, 2001. Copyright 2001, Physicians Postgraduate Press. Reprinted by permission.)

ischaemic heart disease. Modifiable risk factors are diabetes, hypertension, smoking, excessive weight, dyslipidaemia, and physical inactivity. These major risk factors are synergistic, meaning that the total risk of a person suffering a cardiovascular event is more than the sum of the risk conveyed by each major risk factor individually.

Patients with schizophrenia and other psychiatric illnesses are at an increased risk of death from a variety of reasons, including cardiovascular and metabolic causes.[6] In other words, there is an underlying diathesis that renders these patients at greater risk for cardiovascular events than the general population. This likely results from an increased prevalence of cardiac risk factors within this population; they eat less well, smoke more, and take less exercise than the general population, and are more predisposed to obesity and type 2 diabetes.[7–8] Moreover, patients with psychiatric illnesses are less likely than the general population to receive adequate healthcare for comorbid medical conditions, for reasons that are attributed to both the healthcare system and to the nature of the mental illness.[9] For instance, a study by Druss and colleagues,[10] has shown recently that patients with comorbid mental disorders hospitalised for acute myocardial infarction are less than half as likely to receive revascularisation by angioplasty or bypass surgery than patients without a mental illness. Equally concerning is the finding that patients receiving antipsychotic medication are only about 25% as likely to receive lipid-lowering treatments compared with the general population.[11] The increased risk for cardiovascular disease and mortality amongst patients with mental disorders, along with the reduced likelihood of receiving adequate healthcare for comorbid medical conditions, highlights the need for implementation of appropriate primary and secondary preventive measures in this population. The importance of this issue is amplified by concerns regarding the use of some antipsychotic medications which may impart a worse metabolic profile (diabetes, weight gain, increased serum lipid levels) to this already high-risk group of patients.

The novel antipsychotic medications widely used in the management of psychotic disorders, the so-called atypical antipsychotics, represent a major advance in the treatment of schizophrenia, bipolar disorders, psychotic depression, and senile psychoses, among other indications.[12] This class of drugs offers several important advantages over typical antipsychotic drugs, including their characteristic lower risk of extrapyramidal symptoms, in comparison with typical medications at clinically relevant doses.[13] Newer antipsychotics may offer improved treatment of various symptoms, including cognitive impairments associated with the illness, improvements in relapse prevention, and reduced rates of depression and suicidality.[14-17] However, concerns about the cardiovascular adverse effects of the atypical antipsychotic drugs, including the ability to cause weight gain, diabetes and an adverse lipid profile, as well as sudden death due to *torsades de pointes* and other cardiovascular events, have led to concerns about their extensive use.

This chapter reviews the interrelated problems of weight gain, hyperglycaemia, and dyslipidaemia in patients treated with antipsychotic medications. The potential mechanisms for these adverse events are briefly discussed, and suggestions for monitoring and management are outlined. The adverse effects of antipsychotics on cardiac electrophysiology and sudden cardiac death, and myocarditis are reviewed in other chapters.

2. Weight gain

Overweight or obese individuals experience greatly elevated morbidity and mortality from nearly all of the common cardiovascular diseases.[18] Weight gain is also associated with elevated triglyceride levels, diabetes and hypertension, all individual and potent risk factors for cardiovascular disease. Using the 1948 Framingham age and sex distribution data, Fontaine and colleagues[19] estimated the expected impact of weight gain on selected mortality rates amongst adults in the USA. They predicted that for all subjects combined, a mean weight gain of 2.5 kg would be expected to result in an additional 26 to 30 deaths per 100,000 people over 10 years. However in the overweight or obese category (body mass index [BMI] >27 kg/m^2), the same weight gain would be expected to result in an additional 257 to 258 deaths per 100,000 people over 10 years.[19]

There is increasing concern about health issues related to weight gain because of emerging evidence linking the use of certain newer antipsychotics with weight increases in excess of that seen with typical antipsychotics, and the subsequent effects of weight gain on health and compliance. This concern is amplified by the higher prevalence of obesity in patients with mental disorders irrespective of drug therapy. Prior to the first release of atypical antipsychotics in the USA, the 1989 National Health Interview Survey data revealed that a significantly greater proportion of female patients with schizophrenia had BMI distributions in the overweight and obese spectrum compared with the general medical population (Figure 1); a trend toward greater BMI was also seen among male schizophrenic patients.[20] The development of significant weight gain during atypical antipsychotic treatment may further compromise patient health by contributing to comorbid conditions associated with obesity, such as hypertension, coronary artery disease, and type 2 diabetes mellitus.

Over the past few years, a number of articles have been published reviewing the relative weight gain from antipsychotic therapy and imploring action on behalf of the mental health community in the management of this important adverse effect.[21–24] The degree of weight gain associated with extended treatment varies with the agent used, with published studies showing relatively less weight gain with ziprasidone and risperidone, and more substantial gains with the dibenzodiazepine-derived agents, quetiapine, clozapine, and olanzapine. Long-term data with clozapine and olanzapine treated patients reveal weight gain far in excess of that seen with the low-potency typical antipsychotics, such as chlorpromazine or thioridazine. A meta-analysis by Allison and colleagues,[21] estimated body weight gain at 10 weeks associated with atypical antipsychotic use at a standard dose (Figure 2). Estimates of bodyweight gain were statistically significant for clozapine (4.45 kg), olanzapine (4.15 kg), sertindole (2.92 kg), and risperidone (2.1 kg), while that for ziprasidone (0.04 kg) was not

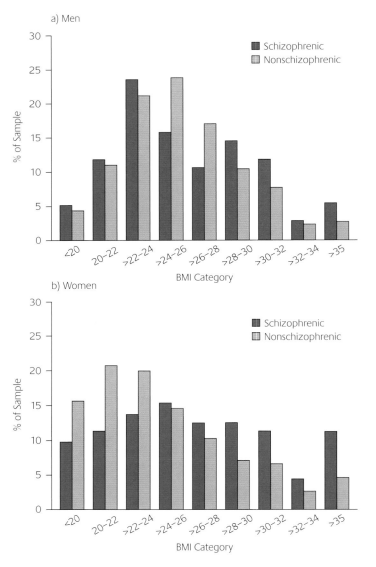

Figure 1. Age-adjusted BMI distribution among schizophrenic and non-schizophrenic individuals in the 1989 National Health Interview Survey.

(Reprinted from Ref 20. Allison DB. The distribution of body mass index among individuals with and without schizophrenia. *J Clinical Psychiatry* 60; 4: 215–220, 1999. Copyright 1999, Physicians Postgraduate Press. Reprinted by permission.)

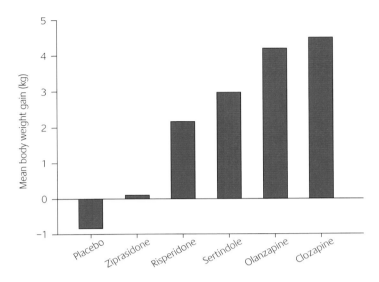

Figure 2. Estimated mean weight gain after 10 weeks' treatment with standard dosages of atypical antipsychotics.

(Adapted from Ref 21 with permission. *Am J Psychiatry* 156: 11, 1686–1696, 1999. Copyright 1999 the American Psychiatric Association; http://ajp.psychiatryonline.org. Reprinted by permission.)

estimated to differ from placebo.[21] Quetiapine also seems to be associated with significant weight gain compared with placebo. In a comparative study, body weight gain in quetiapine-treated patients (average 2 kg) was significantly greater than that with either haloperidol (0.3 kg) or placebo (−0.8 kg), with 16% of patients receiving quetiapine, 4% receiving haloperidol, and 6% receiving placebo, gaining ≥7% of baseline body weight.[25]

The time course of weight gain also seems to vary depending on the agent used, and the potential of each individual agent to cause weight gain. For those atypicals associated with greater weight gain, namely olanzapine and clozapine, a plateau appears between 39 and 52 weeks of therapy, although patients on clozapine treatment may continue to gain approximately 1.8 kg per year for 4 years of treatment.[26–27] In patients receiving ziprasidone, risperidone or quetiapine, the plateau occurs much earlier, typically during the first few months of treatment.[21,22–28] A number of long-term studies have also examined the correlation between weight gain and antipsychotic dosage; the results of these studies suggest that there is no strong association between the two when examined at one year or greater, although shorter term effects cannot be excluded.[26,27]

A number of patient variables have been identified as risk factors that may predict excessive weight gain independent of the particular antipsychotic agent. For instance, a low pretreatment BMI (<23 kg/m^2) is thought to be a significant predictor of weight gain in some studies. Combined data from four separate studies of 2,418 patients treated with olanzapine revealed that a significant weight gain (>7% baseline weight) was experienced by 32% of underweight, 18% normal body weight, and 11% of overweight individuals.[29] Some studies have found an increased prevalence of weight gain associated with the use of atypical antipsychotics amongst women and younger patients, although subsequent investigations have not corroborated these findings.[24] The concurrent use of mood stabilisers has also been associated with excessive weight gain. In a retrospective analysis of metabolic adverse effects in patients treated with atypical antipsychotics, concurrent use of lithium or valproate, which themselves have significant potential for weight gain, resulted in twice the amount of weight gain in patients receiving risperidone compared with those who were not taking one of these mood stabilisers, while olanzapine-treated patients taking concurrent lithium or valproate sustained a mean weight gain of 12.3 kg, i.e. almost three times that without these mood stabilisers.[30]

A number of studies have positively correlated weight gain associated with the use of certain atypical antipsychotics (clozapine, risperidone, sulpiride, olanzapine, and zotepine) with clinical improvement.[24,31] On the other hand, the excessive weight gain resulting from the use of atypical antipsychotics can greatly affect a patient's quality of life, due to increased comorbid medical illness, an increased relapse rate associated with non-compliance, or the social stigma associated with being obese[32] (Table 2). Obese patients are 13 times more likely to request discontinuation of their antipsychotic medication because of concerns about weight gain, and three times more likely to be non-compliant with treatment compared with non-obese patients.[33]

Table 2. Consequences of antipsychotic-induced weight gain.

Health risks
    Hypertension
    Atherosclerosis
    Type 2 diabetes
    Cardiovascular disease
    Stroke
Stigmatisation
Non-compliance
Impairment of quality of life
Social withdrawal

(Adapted from Ref 52. Kurzthaler I, Fleischhacker WW. The clinical implications of weight gain in schizophrenia. *J Clin Psychiatry* 62 [Suppl 7]: 32–37, 2001. Copyright 2001, Physicians Postgraduate Press. Reprinted by permission.)

2.1 Mechanisms of antipsychotic-induced weight gain

The mechanisms underlying weight gain associated with the use of atypical antipsychotics are likely to be multifactorial, and are not completely understood. Possible mechanisms include: (i) sedation resulting in a lowering of basal metabolic rate; (ii) decreased caloric utilisation; and (iii) increased thirst and appetite as a result of anticholinergic effects.[34]

Most of the existing data describing the mechanisms of antipsychotic-induced weight gain have emphasised changes in putative neurological pathways hypothesised to participate in increased energy intake (e.g. increased appetite). Much attention has been focused on the role of monoamines at the level of the hypothalamus.[35] Serotonin (5-hydroxytryptamine, 5-HT) is a well known satiety factor which has been implicated in the mechanism of weight gain associated with the use of atypical antipsychotics. Increased serotonin levels at diverse receptors has been shown to decrease feeding behaviour, while antagonism of serotonin stimulates increased energy intake.[36] The specific serotonin receptor involved is thought to be the $5-HT_{2C}$ receptor, which is implicated in hyperphagia and the subsequent development of obesity and adult-onset diabetes.[37] $5-HT_{2C}$ receptors are antagonised by the atypical antipsychotics and other agents, such as tricyclic antidepressants (TCAs), that produce weight gain, and are minimally affected by agents such as haloperidol that produce very little weight gain. In addition, drugs that act as agonists at $5-HT_{2C}$ receptors, such as dexfenfluramine, decrease appetite and are effective weight-loss agents.[38] However, an analysis by Wirshing and colleagues[28] failed to correlate weight gain from clozapine, olanzapine, risperidone, haloperidol, and sertindole with $5\text{-}HT_{2C}$ affinity. Furthermore, ziprasidone which imparts minimal weight gain has been shown to exhibit high *in vivo* affinity for the $5\text{-}HT_{2C}$ receptor. Taken together, these data do not conclusively support a role for serotoninergic pathways in mediating excess weight gain.

Another mechanism postulated to mediate antipsychotic-induced weight gain involves histamine signalling in the hypothalamus. Antagonism of the histamine H_1 receptor has been suggested as the primary mechanism underlying antipsychotic-induced weight gain.[35] Agents with high affinity for central H_1 receptors, including antidepressants, antipsychotics, and centrally acting antihistamines such as cyproheptadine, have well established effects on weight gain.[23] Wirshing and colleagues,[28] found a robust correlation between the affinity of novel antipsychotics for the histamine H_1 receptor and antipsychotic-induced weight gain.[22] It is postulated that histamine antagonism stimulates energy intake centrally by increasing appetite, with a resultant positive energy balance.

Limited data from several small studies have also suggested a role for leptin in the development of excess weight gain associated with some antipsychotics. Leptin is a cytokine product of the *ob* gene related to interleukin-6, secreted by white adipose cells to regulate insulin secretion and energy metabolism via receptors in the hypothalamus, adipocytes, and skeletal muscle.[39] Some studies have shown that treatment with clozapine and olanzapine is associated with effects on leptin physiology that are not seen in patients treated with haloperidol. Whether these atypical antipsychotics have direct effects on leptin homeostasis or simply induce elevated leptin levels as a consequence of weight gain and increased adipose mass remain unknown, and is currently the subject of further research that may have future implications for the treatment of obesity.[39]

A number of other mechanisms have also been proposed to play a role in weight gain associated with antipsychotic treatment, and are the subject of current research (reviewed in Ref 35). These include androgens, γ-aminobutyric acid (GABA) neurotransmission, cytokines such as tumour necrosis factor α (TNF-α), and uncoupling proteins.

3. Hyperglycaemia

Diabetes mellitus is a potent risk factor for coronary atherosclerosis that is characterised by disturbances in insulin, carbohydrate and fat metabolism. Heart disease death rates in adults with diabetes are about two to four times higher than that of people without diabetes.[40] Moreover, a progressive relationship between hyperglycaemia and cardiovascular event risk (e.g. myocardial infarction, stroke) begins at plasma glucose levels well below the threshold for diabetes, or even the less severe conditions of impaired fasting glucose and impaired glucose tolerance.[41]

Abnormalities in glucose regulation were first reported in patients with schizophrenia prior to the introduction of antipsychotic medications, with early reports indicating a pattern of insulin resistance in untreated patients.[42] Some other major neuropsychiatric conditions including affective disorders and Alzheimer's disease have also been associated with diabetes. With the introduction of chlorpromazine, there was a striking increase in the prevalence rates of type 2 diabetes in patients with schizophrenia. Phenothiazine treatment was soon observed to contribute to abnormalities in glucose regulation, including reports of aggravation of existing diabetes and new-onset type 2 diabetes mellitus, and the term "phenothiazine diabetes" appeared in the literature.[42] However, this association was not consistently found for all older antipsychotics, with few reports implicating higher-potency agents like haloperidol.

Recent reports indicate a re-emergence of this adverse event in clinical practice and suggest that certain newer antipsychotic medications may have an even greater propensity than chlorpromazine to contribute to the development of diabetes mellitus. These reports indicate that the strength of this association varies across different novel antipsychotics. Hyperglycaemia, exacerbation of existing type 1 and type 2 diabetes, new-onset type 2 diabetes mellitus, and diabetic ketoacidosis (DKA), a severe and potentially fatal metabolic complication, have all been associated with treatment using clozapine, olanzapine, quetiapine, and risperidone (reviewed in Ref 42). The frequency of reported cases is markedly varied across different antipsychotic agents, a fact that cannot be simply explained by the length on the market or number of prescriptions. Thus, the most cases of adverse events such as new-onset diabetes mellitus or DKA have been reported for clozapine and olanzapine. In contrast, there are relatively few reports describing an association between diabetes mellitus and quetiapine or risperidone,[43] and there is only one report for ziprasidone.[44] However, on the basis of case reports alone, it is not clear whether the relatively higher frequency of hyperglycaemic events in association with certain medications reflects more frequent or larger effects on glucoregulation, or merely a reporting bias.

In most reported cases, hyperglycaemia does not seem to be dose dependent, and is reversible on cessation of treatment with clozapine and olanzapine, and reappears with the reintroduction of these agents. In these reports, the time to occurrence of glucoregulatory disturbances has ranged from 10 days to 18 months, with an average of three months.[42] It also seems that there is a clear difference in time to emergence of adverse effects on glucose metabolism between different antipsychotics, with hyperglycaemia taking twice as long to occur in patients treated with olanzapine than in those treated with clozapine.[45]

In order to accurately identify the true incidence of diabetes mellitus associated with different antipsychotics, and to identify specific groups of individuals at increased risk, epidemiological studies in a large sample of individuals are needed. In the absence of such large scale studies, estimates of the incidence of new-onset diabetes during clozapine and olanzapine treatment, based on small samples of patients, have ranged from 12% to 36% for clozapine, and from 6% to 35% for olanzapine.[46] Similar estimates for the incidence of diabetes associated with other novel antipsychotics are not available.

Further information on the relative risk for hyperglycaemia associated with the use of atypical antipsychotics comes from smaller studies in which sensitive and reliable techniques are used to characterise disturbances in glucose metabolism. In a recent study by Newcomer and colleagues,[47] modified oral glucose tolerance tests were performed in 48 patients with schizophrenia receiving novel antipsychotics, or typical antipsychotics, and 31 untreated healthy controls. Plasma was sampled at different times for measurement of fasting and postload plasma glucose and insulin levels. Subjects with diabetes were excluded, and groups were matched for age and BMI. Olanzapine-treated patients had significant elevations in postload glucose levels at all time-points in comparison to untreated healthy controls, as well as patients receiving typical antipsychotics (Figure 3). The results were similar for patients treated with clozapine, with the additional finding that mean glucose levels continued to rise at the 75-minute measurement. There were no significant differences between patients receiving typical antipsychotics and controls at any time-points. Risperidone-treated patients had similar elevations in postload glucose levels, but these differences were significant only in comparison to untreated healthy controls. When plasma insulin levels were examined, the mean for patients receiving clozapine and olanzapine was significantly higher than that of those receiving haloperidol and controls at 75 minutes (Figure 3), suggesting that the effects of these antipsychotics are primarily on insulin resistance, rather than insulin secretion. The results of this study indicate that certain new antipsychotics are associated with adverse effects on glucose regulation, which can vary in severity and is independent of adiposity.[47]

Most recently, a large retrospective case-control study examined the incidence of diabetes amongst 19,637 patients diagnosed with and treated for schizophrenia.[48] In this population olanzapine was associated with the highest adjusted odds ratio for the development of diabetes (4.4, 95% CI 1.8 – 11.0). However, this risk estimate was based on only nine incident cases. In contrast, treatment with conventional antipsychotics was associated with 268 incident cases of diabetes, but the frequency of prescription meant that the adjusted odds ratio was only 1.3 (95% CI 1.1 – 1.6).

3.1 Mechanisms of antipsychotic-induced hyperglycaemia

Increased resistance to actions of insulin as well as decreased insulin secretion due to decreased β-cell function are involved in the underlying pathophysiology of type 2 diabetes mellitus.[41] A few controlled studies have employed homeostatic model assessment (HOMA), or minimal model assessment to assess insulin resistance and β-cell function using fasting glucose and insulin concentrations. These studies have reported significant increases in insulin resistance in patients treated with olanzapine and clozapine compared with patients receiving typical antipsychotics. These results suggest that the effect of these antipsychotics is due to increased insulin resistance rather than

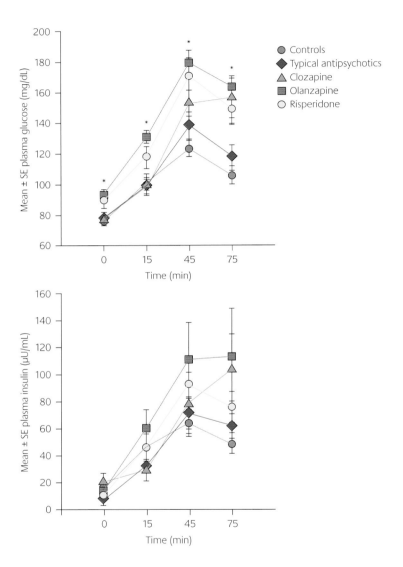

Figure 3. Fasting and postload plasma glucose and insulin levels following a modified oral glucose tolerance test in patients treated with antipsychotics. *$P<0.05$, †$P<0.10$.

(Reprinted from Ref 46. Haupt DW, Newcomer JW. Hyperglycemia and Antipsychotic Medications. *J Clinical Psychiatry* 62 [Suppl 27]: 15–26, 2001. Copyright 2001, Physicians Postgraduate Press. Reprinted by permssion.)

a primary defect in insulin secretion (reviewed in Ref 46). Insulin resistance can develop due to abnormalities at any step in the signalling pathway, including alterations in insulin receptor kinetics and signalling mechanisms. Atypical antipsychotics may induce insulin resistance directly at the insulin receptor site by altering binding characteristics, or interfere with transporter translocation from the microsome to the plasma membrane.[46]

It is also possible that insulin resistance during antipsychotic treatment may arise directly from the effect of these drugs on body weight. Increased abdominal adiposity is well known to increase insulin resistance and contribute to hyperglycaemia and diabetes.[49] The concept that antipsychotic-induced weight gain is directly responsible for treatment related hyperglycaemia is supported by the apparently higher frequency of reported cases of diabetes during treatment with agents that are also associated with more weight gain (clozapine and olanzapine). However, weight gain may not always be required for the development of hyperglycaemia. In an analysis of 45 published cases of new-onset diabetes and DKA associated with atypical antipsychotics, Jin and colleagues[50] found that half the patients manifested no weight gain at the time they presented with diabetes or DKA, although 84% were overweight at the start of antipsychotic treatment. Moreover, studies that have shown diverse effects of different antipsychotics on glucose metabolism, when the groups are matched for BMI, argue against a role for treatment-induced weight gain in development of insulin resistance.[46] Currently, the exact contribution of antipsychotic-induced weight gain to the development of hyperglycaemia remains incompletely understood.

Serotonin receptor activity has also been implicated in regulation of glucose metabolism, with both 5-HT_{1A} and 5-HT_2 receptors implicated.[51] Olanzapine and clozapine both have markedly increased binding affinity to 5-HT_{1A}, 5-HT_{2A}, and 5-HT_{2C} receptors compared with haloperidol and other conventional antipsychotics, with greater affinity for the $5\text{-HT}_{2A/C}$ receptor.[42] The 5-HT_{1A} and 5-HT_{2A} serotonin receptors may have opposing effects on glucose homeostasis. For example, agonism at the 5-HT_{1A} receptors decreases blood glucose levels, whereas antagonism produces hyperglycaemia through decreased pancreatic β-cell responsiveness to blood sugar levels.[52] It is possible that this effect might be sufficient to induce diabetes in predisposed individuals. $5\text{-HT}_{2A/C}$ receptors appear to have effects opposite to those of 5-HT$_{1A}$ receptors in glucose homeostasis. It is therefore difficult to predict the outcome of the simultaneous antagonism of 5-HT$_{1A}$ and 5-HT$_{2A/C}$ receptors that occurs with atypical antipsychotics. Moreover, the rank order of *in vitro* affinities of relevant antipsychotics for serotonin does not fit well with the rank order of their effects on glucose regulation. Consequently, any serotoninergic link between atypical antipsychotics and hyperglycaemia remains speculative.

4. Hyperlipidaemia

An abnormal lipid profile has long been known to increase the risk of coronary artery disease. More recently, elevated triglyceride levels have been identified as an independent risk factor for development of coronary artery disease.[53] An association between antipsychotic drug therapy and hypertriglyceridaemia was first noted after the introduction of typical antipsychotics. Phenothiazines were reported to elevate serum triglyceride and total cholesterol levels, but with greater effects on triglyceride concentrations, while butyrophenones exerted a minimal or slightly favourable effect on serum lipid levels in patients with schizophrenia.[54]

More recently, there have been reports of deranged lipid profiles associated with the use of atypical antipsychotics. It appears that the atypicals exerting the most significant effects on triglyceride levels are the dibenzodiazepine-derived compounds clozapine, olanzapine and quetiapine. Spivak and colleagues,[55] compared a cohort of patients taking clozapine with a similar group on typical antipsychotics for at least one year. They found significant hypertriglyceridaemia in the clozapine group (mean ± SD = 202.9 ± 131.1 mg/dL or 2.3 ± 1.5 mM/L) but not the typical group (134.4 ± 51.9 mg/dL or 1.5 ± 0.6 mM/L), without significant differences in total cholesterol levels. Similar elevations in fasting triglyceride levels have been reported in patients on olanzapine therapy without significant effects on cholesterol levels.[56–57] In a recent retrospective study, Meyer[58] reported 14 cases of severe hypertriglyceridaemia (>600 mg/dL or 6.8 mM/L) associated with olanzapine and quetiapine therapy. Much less of an effect on serum lipids is observed with other novel antipsychotics. In a retrospective study, olanzapine treated patients experienced significantly greater increases in fasting triglyceride levels at one year (+104.8 mg/dL or 1.2 mM/L) compared with those on risperidone (+31.7 mg/dL or 0.4 mM/L), with similarly increased effects on cholesterol levels (+30.7 vs +7.2 mg/dL or 0.8 vs 0.2 mM/L).[30] Moreover, patients switched from olanzapine to ziprasidone were shown to have a significant decrease in serum triglyceride and cholesterol levels over a period of six weeks.[59]

Some studies have reported a significant association between weight gain and changes in triglyceride levels in patients receiving atypical antipsychotic therapy, thereby suggesting that hypertriglyceridaemia may be secondary to increased weight gain.[26,56] Other studies, however, have not found a similar correlation between antipsychotic-induced weight gain and hypertriglyceridaemia, raising the possibility that some atypical antipsychotics may have direct effects on serum lipid levels.[58–60] In a retrospective analysis comparing metabolic outcomes during the first year of treatment with risperidone or olanzapine, Meyer showed comparable weight gain for both agents (3.7 vs 4.6 kg respectively), but the olanzapine group experienced a mean increase in serum triglyceride levels of 84.8 mg/dL (1.0 mM/L) compared with a 20.2 mg/dL (0.2 mM/L) increase for the risperidone cohort. Furthermore, a study examining the cardiovascular risk of olanzapine and risperidone that had matched the two cohorts for BMI, found that 32% of the olanzapine group compared with 5% of the risperidone group manifested the atherogenic metabolic triad of hyperinsulinaemia, elevated apolipoprotein B, and small dense LDL concentrations.[60] It has also been reported that patients switched from olanzapine to ziprasidone experienced a significant decrease in serum triglyceride and cholesterol levels over six weeks, despite average weight loss of only 1.5 kg.

It appears that the atypicals exerting the most significant effects on fasting triglyceride levels are the dibenzodiazepine-derived compounds. The mechanisms by which these atypical antipsychotics exert their influence on triglyceride metabolism are not clearly understood at present.

5. Monitoring and treatment of adverse metabolic effects

Patients on treatment with atypical antipsychotic agents should undergo regular monitoring of their weight, plasma glucose, and cholesterol and triglyceride levels, so that clinicians can individualise treatment decisions and reduce the risks of morbidity and cardiovascular events. Wide individual variations exist in both the timing of derangement in glucose regulation and lipid levels, as well as the magnitude of these metabolic disturbances. This necessitates frequent monitoring of total triglyceride and cholesterol levels, and fasting plasma glucose levels for the first year after the initiation of treatment with any of the atypical antipsychotics. It is also prudent to perform these tests prior to, and after, starting or changing antipsychotic therapy. Monitoring of glucose and lipid levels should be performed in conjunction with weight monitoring due to the additional and independent risk that weight gain poses. An enquiry should be made about the other major risk factors for diabetes and cardiovascular disease; family history of diabetes or ischaemic heart disease, previous diagnosis of gestational diabetes or impaired glucose tolerance, hypertension, and smoking.

The treatment of obesity and changing eating behaviours is challenging in individuals with a major mental illness; nevertheless, there is evidence for success in the behavioural management of obesity in the chronically mentally ill.[24] The essential aspects of any behavioural intervention for overweight or obese individuals comprise frequent monitoring, nutritional and lifestyle counselling geared toward the population, and skills training focusing on exercise, nutrition, health education, and behavioural techniques. Weight loss intervention may also include the option to switch to an antipsychotic that may not cause significant weight gain. Pharmacological therapy with appetite suppressants is generally reserved for obese patients who fail to lose weight with several months of behavioural interventions, particularly those with comorbid conditions such as diabetes.

In patients with hyperglycaemia at levels classified as impaired glucose tolerance or impaired fasting glucose, the mainstay of treatment is a programme of diet and exercise, along with control of triglyceride levels, blood pressure and weight. On the other hand, the diagnosis of frank diabetes usually necessitates treatment with hypoglycaemic agents such as sulphonylureas, biguanides, thiazolidinediones, or insulin, combined with diet and exercise interventions. However, if non-compliance limits the effectiveness of these interventions, or even when optimal management of diabetes is successful, the question remains as to whether the patient could be best served by treatment with an equally effective antipsychotic that does not require intensive medication and lifestyle interventions to maintain normoglycaemia. Early collaboration with the primary care physician, or a general physician, is necessary to integrate difficult decisions about the management of diabetes and hyperglycaemia along with psychiatric treatment decisions.

In patients treated with dibenzodiazepine-derived antipsychotics, a characteristic clinical course is usually seen when serum lipids are serially monitored after the onset of therapy, with peak triglyceride levels typically occurring within the first year, followed by a decrease and subsequent period of stabilisation.[46] In general, patients can be observed without treatment until achieving a period of stabilisation unless the triglyceride levels are severely raised, thereby putting patients at risk for acute pancreatitis. If hypertriglyceridaemia becomes sustained, treatment should be initiated as elevated triglyceride levels are now recognised as an independent risk factor for coronary artery disease. Weight reduction and the use of diets low in saturated fats are considered the mainstays in the treatment of mild triglyceride abnormalities. If these measurements fail, pharmacological therapy is used to achieve direct reductions in serum triglyceride levels. The common agents used include fish oil and fibric acid derivatives. In patients with diabetes, established cardiovascular disease and/or coincident hypercholesterolaemia, a statin would be the agent of choice for treating hypertriglyceridaemia. However, the effects of statins on triglyceride levels are relatively modest, so that the subsequent addition of fish oil or fibric acid derivatives may still be necessary. Liaison with a general physician or lipid clinic would be beneficial.

6. Conclusions

Patients with major psychiatric disorders suffer increased morbidity and mortality due to cardiovascular disease, with presumed contributions from a number of modifiable risk factors such as smoking, sedentary lifestyle, poor diet, obesity, hyperglycaemia, and dyslipidaemia. Some of these risk factors may be difficult for patients to modify on their own, and potential iatrogenic contributions to cardiovascular risk have understandably come under increasing scrutiny.

The novel antipsychotic agents represent a major advance in the treatment of schizophrenia, bipolar disorders, psychotic depression, and senile psychoses, among other indications. These agents have produced dramatic improvements in the treatment of psychoses, including reduced incidence of extrapyramidal effects, better control of the positive symptoms of psychosis, improved cognition, less depression, and reduced suicidality. However, there is also increasing evidence that some atypical antipsychotic drugs adversely affect the patients' metabolic profile with resultant weight gain, hyperglycaemia and increases in lipids. These, as well as reports of sudden death due to *torsades de pointes* and other cardiovascular events associated with the use of atypical antipsychotics, have led to concerns about their extensive use.

It is important that clinicians, in conjunction with patients and their family members, balance the significant benefits of atypical antipsychotic treatment against the risk of metabolic disturbances and select an appropriate course of treatment specific to the individual patient. This should include a regular program of monitoring for adverse metabolic and cardiovascular effects, with increased awareness of possible metabolic changes during atypical antipsychotic treatment, and early recognition of the need for behavioural and pharmacological therapeutic intervention, or a switch to different antipsychotic therapy. It is also important for psychiatrists to build a close working relationship with the general physician or the general practitioner with an interest in diabetes. Such a treatment strategy would encourage a regular assessment of the overall medical needs of the psychiatric patient, and may reduce the anxiety associated with the use of a drug when the psychiatric condition clearly indicates that the drug can be of value.

References

1. McGovern PG, Pankow JS, Shahar E, *et al.* Recent trends in acute coronary heart disease: Mortality, morbidity, medical care, and risk factors. The Minnesota Heart Survey Investigators. *N Engl J Med* 1996; **334**: 884–890.

2. Hunink MGM, Goldman L, Tosteson ANA, *et al.* The recent decline in mortality from coronary heart disease, 1980–1990: The effect of secular trends in risk factors and treatment. *JAMA* 1997; **277**: 535–542.

3. Rosengren A, Dotevall A, Eriksson H, *et al.* Optimal risk factors in the population: Prognosis, prevalence, and secular trends; data from Goteborg population studies. *Eur Heart J* 2001; **22**: 136–144.

4. Grundy SM, Balady GJ, Criqui MH, *et al.* Guide to primary prevention of cardiovascular diseases: A statement for healthcare professionals from the Task Force on Risk Reduction. American Heart Association Science Advisory and Coordinating Committee. *Circulation* 1997; **95**: 2329–2331.

5. Wood D, De Backer G, Faergeman O, *et al.* Prevention of coronary heart disease in clinical practice: Recommendations of the Second Joint Task Force of European and

other Societies on Coronary Prevention. *Atherosclerosis* 1998; **140**: 199–270.

6. Harris EC, Barraclough B. Excess mortality of mental disorder. *Br J Psychiatry* 1998; **173**: 11–53.

7. Brown S, Birtwistle J, Roe L, *et al.* The unhealthy lifestyle of people with schizophrenia. *Psychol Med* 1999; **29**: 697–701.

8. Brown S, Inskip H, Barraclough B. Causes of the excess mortality of schizophrenia. *Br J Psychiatry* 2000; **177**: 212–217.

9. Goldman LS. Medical illness in patients with schizophrenia. *J Clin Psychiatry* 1999; **60**: 10–15.

10. Druss BG, Bradford DW, Rosenheck RA, *et al.* Mental disorders and use of cardiovascular procedures after myocardial infarction. *JAMA* 2000; **283**: 506–511.

11. Redelmeier DA, Tan SH, Booth GL. The treatment of unrelated disorders in patients with chronic medical diseases. *N Engl J Med* 1998; **338**: 1516–1520.

12. Casey DE. Side effect profiles of new antipsychotic agents. *J Clin Psychiatry* 1996; **57**: 40–45.

13. Breier AF, Malhotra AK, Su T-P, *et al.* Clozapine and risperidone in chronic schizophrenia: Effects on symptoms, parkinsonian side effects, and neuroendocrine response. *Am J Psychiatry* 1999; **156**: 294–298.

14. Meltzer HY, Okayli G. Reduction of suicidality during clozapine treatment of neuroleptic-resistant schizophrenia: Impact on risk-benefit assessment. *Am J Psychiatry* 1995; **152**: 183–190.

15. Collaborative Working Group on Clinical Trial Evaluation. Evaluating the effects of antipsychotics on cognition in schizophrenia. *J Clin Psychiatry* 1998; **59(Suppl 12)**: 35–40.

16. Keefe RS, Silva SG, Perkins DO, *et al.* The effects of atypical antipsychotic drugs on neurocognitive impairment in schizophrenia: A review and meta-analysis. *Schizophr Bull* 1999; **25**: 201–222.

17. Tollefson GD, Sanger TM, Lu Y, *et al.* Depressive signs and symptoms in schizophrenia: A prospective blinded trial of olanzapine and haloperidol. *Arch Gen Psychiatry* 1998; **55**: 250–258.

18. Eckel RH, Barouch WW, Ershow AG. Report of the National Heart, Lung, and Blood Institute-National Institute of Diabetes and Digestive and Kidney Diseases Working Group on the pathophysiology of obesity-associated

cardiovascular disease. *Circulation* 2002; **105**: 2923–2928.

19. Fontaine KR, Heo M, Harrigan EP, *et al.* Estimating the consequences of anti-psychotic induced weight gain on health and mortality rate. *Psychiatry Res* 2001; **101**: 277–288.

20. Allison DB, Fontaine KR, Heo M, *et al.* The distribution of body mass index among individuals with and without schizophrenia. *J Clin Psychiatry* 1999; **60**: 215–220.

21. Allison DB, Mentore JL, Heo M, *et al.* Antipsychotic-induced weight gain: A comprehensive research synthesis. *Am J Psychiatry* 1999; **156**: 1686–1696.

22. Taylor DM, McAskill R. Atypical antipsychotics and weight gain – a systematic review. *Acta Psychiatr Scand* 2000; **101**: 416–432.

23. Sussman N. Review of atypical antipsychotics and weight gain. *J Clin Psychiatry* 2001; **62**: 5–12.

24. Russell JM, Mackell JA. Bodyweight gain associated with atypical antipsychotics: Epidemiology and therapeutic implications. *CNS Drugs* 2001; **15**: 537–551.

25. Arvanitis LA, Miller BG. The Seroquel Trial 13 Study Group. Multiple fixed doses of "Seroquel" (quetiapine) in patients with acute exacerbation of schizophrenia: A comparison with haloperidol and placebo. *Biol Psychiatry* 1997; **42**: 233–246.

26. Henderson DC, Cagliero E, Gray C, *et al.* Clozapine, diabetes mellitus, weight gain, and lipid abnormalities: A five-year naturalistic study. *Am J Psychiatry* 2000; **157**: 975–981.

27. Kinon BJ, Basson BR, Gilmore JA, *et al.* Long-term olanzapine treatment: Weight change and weight-related health factors in schizophrenia. *J Clin Psychiatry* 2001; **62**: 92–100.

28. Wirshing DA, Wirshing WC, Kysar L, *et al.* Novel antipsychotics: Comparison of weight gain liabilities. *J Clin Psychiatry* 1999; **60**: 358–363.

29. Beasley CM, Jr., Tollefson GD, Tran PV. Safety of olanzapine. *J Clin Psychiatry* 1997; **58(Suppl 10)**: 13–17.

30. Meyer JM. A retrospective comparison of weight, lipid, and glucose changes between risperidone- and olanzapine-treated inpatients: Metabolic outcomes after 1 year. *J Clin Psychiatry* 2002; **63**: 425–433.

31. Czobor P, Volavka J, Sheitman B, *et al.* Antipsychotic-induced weight gain and

therapeutic response: A differential association. *J Clin Psychopharmacol* 2002; **22**: 244–251.

32. Kurzthaler I, Fleischhacker WW. The clinical implications of weight gain in schizophrenia. *J Clin Psychiatry* 2001; **62**: 32–37.

33. Weiden PJ, Allison DB, Mackell JA. Obesity as risk factor of antipsychotic noncompliance. In: New Research Abstracts of the 153rd Annual Meeting of the American Psychiatric Association; May 18, 2000; Chicago, IL. Abstract NR218: 114.

34. Masand PS. Weight gain associated with psychotropic drugs. *Expert Opin Pharmacother* 2000; **1**: 377–389.

35. McIntyre RS, Mancini DA, Basile VS. Mechanisms of antipsychotic-induced weight gain. *J Clin Psychiatry* 2001; **62**: 23–29.

36. De Vry J, Schreiber R. Effects of selected serotonin 5-HT(1) and 5-HT(2) receptor agonists on feeding behavior: Possible mechanisms of action. *Neurosci Biobehav Rev* 2000; **24**: 341–353.

37. Tecott LH, Sun LM, Akana SF, *et al*. Eating disorder and epilepsy in mice lacking 5-HT$_{2C}$ serotonin receptors. *Nature* 1995; **374**: 542–546.

38. Rissanen A. Pharmacological intervention: The antiobesity approach. *Eur J Clin Invest* 1998; **28(Suppl 2)**: 27–30.

39. Mantzoros CS. The role of leptin in human obesity and disease: A review of current evidence. *Ann Intern Med* 1999; **130**: 671–680.

40. Mak KH, Topol EJ. Emerging concepts in the management of acute myocardial infarction in patients with diabetes mellitus. *J Am Coll Cardiol* 2000; **35**: 563–568.

41. Taegtmeyer H, McNulty P, Young ME. Adaptation and maladaptation of the heart in diabetes: Part I: general concepts. *Circulation* 2002; **105**: 1727–1733.

42. Lindenmayer JP, Nathan AM, Smith RC. Hyperglycemia associated with the use of atypical antipsychotics. *J Clin Psychiatry* 2001; **62**: 30–38.

43. Goodnick PJ, Kato MM. Antipsychotic medication: Effects on regulation of glucose and lipids. *Expert Opin Pharmacother* 2001; **2**: 1571–1582.

44. Yang SH, McNeely MJ. Rhabdomyolysis, pancreatitis, and hyperglycemia with ziprasidone. *Am J Psychiatry* 2002; **159**: 1435.

45. Mir S, Taylor D. Atypical antipsychotics and hyperglycaemia. *Int Clin Psychopharmacol* 2001; **16**: 63–73.

46. Haupt DW, Newcomer JW. Hyperglycemia and antipsychotic medications. *J Clin Psychiatry* 2001; **62**: 15–26.

47. Newcomer JW, Haupt DW, Fucetola R, *et al*. Abnormalities in glucose regulation during antipsychotic treatment of schizophrenia. *Arch Gen Psychiatry* 2002; **59**: 337–345.

48. Koro CE, Fedder DO, L'Italien GJ, *et al*. Assessment of independent effect of olanzapine and risperidone on risk of diabetes among patients with schizophrenia: Population based nested case-control study. *BMJ* 2002; **325**: 243.

49. Reaven G. Metabolic syndrome: Pathophysiology and implications for management of cardiovascular disease. *Circulation* 2002; **106**: 286–288.

50. Jin H, Meyer JM, Jeste DV. Phenomenology of and risk factors for new-onset diabetes mellitus and diabetic ketoacidosis associated with atypical antipsychotics: An analysis of 45 published cases. *Ann Clin Psychiatry* 2002; **14**: 59–64.

51. Wirshing DA, Spellberg BJ, Erhart SM, *et al*. Novel antipsychotics and new onset diabetes. *Biol Psychiatry* 1998; **44**: 778–783.

52. Uvnas-Moberg K, Ahlenius S, Alster P, *et al*. Effects of selective serotonin and dopamine agonists on plasma levels of glucose, insulin and glucagon in the rat. *Neuroendocrinology* 1996; **63**: 269–274.

53. Assmann G, Schulte H, Funke H, *et al*. The emergence of triglycerides as a significant independent risk factor in coronary artery disease. *Eur Heart J* 1998; **19(Suppl M)**: M8–14.

54. Arana GW. An overview of side effects caused by typical antipsychotics. *J Clin Psychiatry* 2000; **61**: 5–11.

55. Spivak B, Roitman S, Vered Y, *et al*. Diminished suicidal and aggressive behavior, high plasma norepinephrine levels, and serum triglyceride levels in chronic neuroleptic-resistant schizophrenic patients maintained on clozapine. *Clin Neuropharmacol* 1998; **21**: 245–250.

56. Osser DN, Najarian DM, Dufresne RL. Olanzapine increases weight and serum triglyceride levels. *J Clin Psychiatry* 1999; **60**: 767–770.

57. Sheitman BB, Bird PM, Binz W, *et al*. Olanzapine-induced elevation of plasma

triglyceride levels. *Am J Psychiatry* 1999; **156**: 1471–1472.

58. Meyer JM. Novel antipsychotics and severe hyperlipidemia. *J Clin Psychopharmacol* 2001; **21**: 369–374.

59. Kingsbury SJ, Fayek M, Trufasiu D, *et al*. The apparent effects of ziprasidone on plasma lipids and glucose. *J Clin Psychiatry* 2001; **62**: 347–349.

60. Bouchard RH, Demers MF, Simoneau I, *et al*. Atypical antipsychotics and cardiovascular risk in schizophrenic patients. *J Clin Psychopharmacol* 2001; **21**: 110–111.

Effects of antipsychotic drugs on the autonomic nervous system: Orthostatic hypotension and syncope

A. John Camm and Irina Savelieva

Department of Cardiological Sciences, St George's Hospital Medical School

London, United Kingdom

Correspondence: Professor A. John Camm, MD, FRCP,

Professor of Clinical Cardiology, Department of

Cardiological Sciences,

St. George's Hospital Medical School,

Cranmer Terrace, London, SW17 0RE.

Telephone: +44 (0)20 8725 3554 Facsimile: +44 (0)20 8767 7141

Email: jcamm@sghms.ac.uk

1. Introduction

The ideal antipsychotic drug would be one that provides a beneficial effect on the mental disorder being treated but produces no unwanted side-effects on other systems. All antipsychotic agents that are currently available are known to cause a wide range of pathophysiologic responses, including specific cardiovascular effects, and these potential effects are of continuing clinical concern. Retrospective studies have shown that cardiovascular mortality in psychiatric patients is higher than in the general population, particularly in patients receiving antipsychotics to treat schizophrenia.[1-4] There is increasing evidence of a disproportionate number of sudden deaths in psychiatric patients taking antipsychotic drugs which cannot be attributed to unrecognised suicide, accident proneness, or co-existing substance misuse.[4-5] A review of in-patient mortality in five psychiatric hospitals over 12 years has identified 1,350 deaths, and 74 (5.5%) of these were unexplained sudden deaths.[6] Fatal ventricular tachyarrhythmias associated with QT interval prolongation (most often *torsades de pointes*), malignant hypotension and bradycardia resulting in cardiorespiratory arrest, have been implicated in the genesis of sudden death in this clinical setting.[7–9] This review will (i) discuss the evidence from observational and premarketing clinical randomised studies on the incidence and clinical relevance of orthostatic hypotension and syncope in patients receiving antipsychotic treatment; (ii) outline multiple receptor blockades as they pertain to the cardiovascular effects of antipsychotic drugs; and (iii) compare the propensity of individual agents to impede autonomic nervous system regulation.

2. Pathophysiologic mechanisms of autonomic effects of antipsychotic drugs

The net effect of antipsychotic drugs on the autonomic nervous system is the result of complex interactions between multiple receptor agonism and antagonism. All antipsychotics exhibit a high affinity for numerous receptors, including dopaminergic (D_1–D_4), serotonergic (5-HT receptor subtypes), histaminergic (H_1), α_1 and α_2-adrenergic, muscarinic (M_1, M_2), and GABAergic (gamma-aminobutyric acid) as a part of their pharmacologic spectrum.

2.1 Adrenergic receptors

The α-adrenoblocking properties of antipsychotic drugs have long been associated with the origin of orthostatic hypotension in psychiatric patients. The net effect on the peripheral vascular tone of α_1- and α_2-adrenoreceptor blockade depends on the localisation of the receptors.[10] The blockade of α_1-and α_2-adrenoreceptors at postsynaptic sites results in peripheral vasodilatation and a decrease in systemic blood pressure, whereas the blockade of presynaptic α_2-adrenoreceptors produces the opposite effect by enhancing the presynaptic release of norepinephrine which in its turn activates postsynaptic α- and β-receptors, thus causing vasoconstriction and tachycardia. The blockade of α_2-adrenoreceptors in certain regions of the central nervous system, such as the nucleus tractus solitarius, vagal nucleus, and vasomotor centre, causes the reduction in peripheral sympathetic nervous system activity and augments vagal stimulation, resulting in peripheral vasodilatation and bradycardia.

Some antipsychotic agents (e.g. risperidone) have been shown to exert weak β-adrenoreceptor antagonism. The presynaptic blockade of β_2-receptors reduces the rate of norepinephrine release from presynaptic storage. Alternatively, the ability of antipsychotic drugs to block postsynaptic β_1-receptors results in the inhibition of neuronal re-uptake of norepinephrine. The net effect is reduced cardiac contractility and bradycardia. β-adrenoreceptors are present in various structures of the central nervous system, but their functional role and potential basis as a therapeutic target remain uncertain. They are probably similar to their peripheral counterparts, as suggested by radioligand-binding experiments. More recently, β_3-adrenoreceptors have been identified in the smooth muscle cells of blood vessels but their role in regulating vascular tone has not yet been defined.

2.2 Muscarinic receptors

There are five genetic (m_1–m_5) and four pharmacologic (M_1–M_4) subtypes of muscarinic receptors, which are heterogeneous with regard to regional distribution, primary effector mechanisms, and function.[11–12] The central nervous system also contains muscarinic receptors which are probably involved in the central regulation of blood pressure and heart rate. Muscarinic receptors have been also demonstrated in peripheral sympathetic neurons. The stimulation of M_1-muscarinic receptors located in the central nervous system has been shown to evoke vasopressor and cardioacceleratory responses that are inhibited by the selective M_1-receptor antagonist, pirenzepine.[13] Central M_1-receptor activation is also involved in mediating the Bezold-Jarisch reflex.[14] Experimental studies suggest that the vasopressor effects of central M_1-receptor stimulation on increased sympathetic outflow may be mediated by the stimulation of α_1-receptors in the nucleus tractus solitarius, or through 5-HT-receptors in the posterior hypothalamus.[15–16] Thus, alterations in M_1-receptor activity in the brain may influence autonomic nervous system control of cardiovascular function.

Many antipsychotic agents are potent muscarinic receptor blockers. Anticholinergic effects on the heart are mediated through M_2-muscarinic receptor blockade, resulting in vagal inhibition and tachycardia which is usually modest in the absence of sympathetic stimulation. M_1-receptor blockade in the central nervous system by antipsychotic drugs may result in diminishing cardioacceleratory and vasopressor effects usually realising through central M_1-receptor activity. M_1-receptor blockade in the sympathetic ganglia is associated with presynaptic feedback inhibition of norepinephrine release by acetylcholine, thus contributing to peripheral vasodilatation and hypotension caused by α-adrenoblockade.

There is experimental evidence that the blockade of vascular M_3-muscarinic receptors may reduce the release of the endothelium-derived relaxant factor (EDRF), assumed to function like nitric oxide, an important endogenous vasodilator agent, and consequently, may cause peripheral vasoconstriction.

2.3 Serotonin receptors

At present, at least seven types of serotonin (5-HT) receptors have been identified, and each of these classes consists of multiple subtypes. Due to the great diversity of serotonin receptors, a single neurotransmitter may produce a vide variety of cellular effects in multiple neuronal systems. Serotonin has been implicated in baroreflex modulation at the level of the nucleus tractus solitarius, and both inhibitory and excitatory control of sympathetic preganglionic neurons via the different receptor subtypes.[10]

Experimental studies have provided evidence that central 5-HT containing pathways implicated in cardiovascular regulation involve two major receptor subtypes: 5-HT_{1A} and 5-HT_{2A}.[17-18] Activation of 5-HT_2-receptors, mainly 5-HT_{2A}-subtype in the midbrain, generally mediates sympathetic outflow to the heart and produces hypertension. 5-HT_{2A}- and 5-HT_{2B}-receptor subtypes have also been shown to be responsible for the release of vasopressin by activation of a central angiotensinergic pathway.[19]

Abundant experimental evidence has implicated central 5-HT_{1A}-receptors in the control of the excitability cardiac vagal preganglionic neurons, and subsequently in the reflex regulation of parasympathetic outflow.[18] The stimulation of 5-HT_{1A}-serotonin receptor subtypes causes the inhibition of sympathetic neural outflow and an increase in adrenal sympathetic stimulation, resulting in diminished peripheral vasoconstriction in conjunction with accentuation of adrenal epinephrine release.[20-21] Several antipsychotic agents, clozapine, ziprasidone, and iloperidone, are known to share 5-HT_{1A}-agonistic properties. Ziprasidone has also been shown to decrease synaptic re-intake of serotonin and norepinephrine. There is also some evidence that activation of $5\text{-HT}_{1D/1F}$-receptors can cause centrally mediated hypotension, whereas 5-HT_{1B}-subtype appears to produce an opposite effect.[22]

Finally, 5-HT$_3$-receptors are implicated in the afferent regulation of sympathetic and parasympathetic tone, and are believed to be essential in the pathophysiology of the Bezold-Jarisch reflex.[23-24] The stimulation of 5-HT$_3$-receptors has been shown to inhibit the cardiovagal component of the Bezold-Jarisch reflex without affecting its sympathetic component.

2.4 Histamine receptors

The histaminergic system plays an important pathophysiologic role in cardiovascular regulation. Three histaminic receptor subtypes have been identified. Histamine H$_1$-receptors are expressed in the central nervous system, gastrointestinal tract, and in smooth muscle cells of blood vessel walls. The blockade of H$_1$-histamine receptors at different levels by antipsychotic drugs may provide different effects on peripheral vascular tone. In an experimental study, microinjection of H$_1$-receptor antagonist mepyramine into mesencephalic nucleus dorsalis raphe evoked hypotension and bradycardia.[25] H$_2$-receptors are present in the central nervous system and the heart, and are essential in mediating sympathoinhibitory responses elicited in the rostral ventrolateral medulla.[26]

Unlike H$_1$- and H$_2$-histamine receptors, H$_3$-receptors are located presynaptically both on histaminergic and non-histaminic nerve terminals, where they inhibit the release of a variety of neurotransmitters, thus contributing to regulation of vascular tone.[27] In experimental studies, the stimulation of H$_3$-receptors produced cardioinhibitory and vasodepressor effects.[28]

2.5 Dopamine receptors

Catecholamines in the central nervous system include dopamine, noradrenaline, and adrenaline. Dopamine β-hydroxylase allows transformation of dopamine into noradrenaline. Noradrenaline and adrenaline neurons form two anatomically segregated but functionally integrated systems, and have extensive interconnections with areas involved in autonomic and neurohumoral control of cardiovascular system. Catecholamines have been implicated in both excitatory and inhibitory modulation of preganglionic sympathetic neurons, facilitation of the baroreflex at the level of the nucleus tractus solitarius, and stimulation of vasopressin secretion from the hypothalamus. The responses to catecholamines are complex, and involve excitatory and inhibitory effects mediated through α_1- and α_2-receptors, respectively.

It is widely reported in the literature that the therapeutic efficacy of antipsychotic drugs relates to their affinity to block D_2-dopamine receptors in the central nervous system, whereas the functional role and the primary effector mechanisms of D_1-, D_3-, D_4-, and D_5-dopamine receptor subtypes is less understood. It is plausible that the ability of many antipsychotic agents to block D_2-receptors as well as other dopamine receptor subtypes may account for central and autonomic regulation of peripheral vascular tone.

2.6 GABAergic receptors

GABA is now recognised as the most abundant inhibitory neurotransmitter within the central nervous system, which produces both pre- and postsynaptic inhibition through $GABA_A$- and $GABA_B$-receptors. GABA has been implicated in both tonic and reflex inhibition of medullary vasomotor, cardiovagal, and hypothalamic neurons and is responsible for the vasodepressor effects and bradycardia.[27,29-30] A variety of pharmacologic agents can influence the activity of $GABA_A$-receptors, as at least five separate drug binding sites have been identified, specifically for benzodiazepines and barbiturates. Antipsychotic agents, even with a weak affinity to benzodiazepine receptors (e.g. olanzapine), can exert agonistic effects on $GABA_A$-receptors, thus potentiating their inhibitory action on sympathetic outflow and vasoconstriction. Finally, the hypotensive reactions may be facilitated by inappropriate antidiuretic hormone secretion, a rare toxic effect of antipsychotic therapy.

In summary, the net effect of antipsychotic drugs on the autonomic nervous system and on the development of orthostatic hypotension and bradycardia in particular, is the result of multiple receptor binding at various levels, and the involvement of different neurotransmitters.

3. Orthostatic hypotension

Orthostatic hypotension is the most common and potentially serious autonomic side effect of antipsychotic drugs. Figure 1 shows the prevalence of hypotension and dizziness associated with antipsychotic drugs in clinical trials and observational studies. Transient hypotensive reactions have been noted in up to 75% of patients receiving antipsychotic therapy.[31] A reduction in systolic

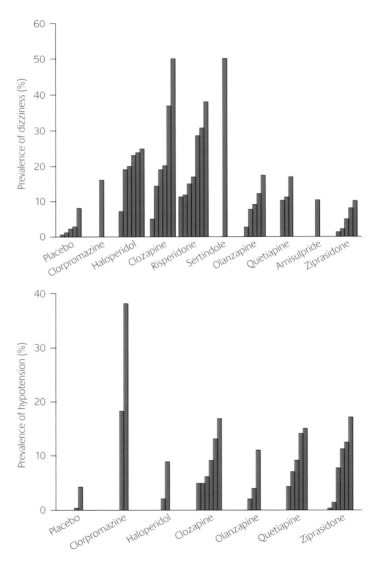

Figure 1. The prevalence of hypotension and dizziness associated with antipsychotic drugs.

blood pressure by 20 mmHg was observed in 77% of 196 patients receiving long-term treatment with chlorpromazine, thioridazine or haloperidol, and a reduction in excess of 40 mmHg was recorded in 11%.[32] Such a reduction in blood pressure persisted during three minutes of the upright posture in 16.8% of patients. Patients receiving a combination of two antipsychotic drugs tended to develop orthostatic hypotension more often compared with those on monotherapy (80.2% vs 71% at 1 minute and 22% vs 6.5% at three minutes). However, from Figure 1 it is clear that orthostatic hypotension and dizziness, which would be expected to be an important symptom of decreased systolic blood pressure, often did not parallel each other and may be regarded as side-effects of antipsychotic drugs related to different systems, e.g. the cardiovascular system (hypotension) and the central nervous system (dizziness). Thus, 19% of 342 patients treated with clozapine were reported to have dizziness, whereas only 9% had an actual drop in systolic blood pressure following postural changes.[33] In a different report on 1,080 patients who participated in premarketing clinical trials of clozapine, the incidence of dizziness or *vertigo* was 5% and so was the incidence of orthostatic hypotension with or without syncope.[33] These observations raise questions as to whether dizziness may be a reliable symptom of postural hypotension, indicating the need for close monitoring of haemodynamics especially at the early stages of treatment, or if it merely relates to specific actions of antipsychotic agents on the central nervous system.

The propensity to affect cardiovascular autonomic status varies largely among the different types of antipsychotic drugs. It is generally greater with low potency (i.e. administered at doses equal or greater than 200 mg/day) typical antipsychotics that predominantly act as dopamine-receptor antagonists, particularly chlorpromazine and thioridazine. Mid- to high-potency agents, for which therapeutic doses range from 2 to 120 mg/day (e.g. haloperidol, fluphenazine, loxapine, molindone), are associated with a lower frequency of severe hypotension. However, certain atypical agents (i.e. deprived of extrapyramidal effects due to a higher affinity to the mesolimbic rather than the striatal dopamine system) with serotonin-dopamine antagonism, particularly clozapine and sertindole, have been reported to produce significant autonomic imbalance (Table 1). The strong cholinergic and α_1-adrenergic antagonistic action of clozapine contributes to autonomic

Table 1. Autonomic Effects of Antipsychotic Drugs

Drug	Autonomic effects due to			
	α_1-adreno-receptor blockade	α_2-adreno-receptor blockade	H_1-histaminic receptor blockade	M_1/M_2-muscarinic receptor blockade
Typical antipsychotics				
Phenothiazines				
Clorpromazine	+++	+++	+++	+++
Thioridazine	+++	+++	+++	+++
Trifluoroperazine	++	+	++	++
Perphenazine	++	+	++	++
Fluphenazine	+	+	+	+
Thioxanthenes				
Thiothixene	++	+	++	++
Flupenthixol	++	+	++	++
Zuclopenthixol	++	+	++	++
Diphenylbutyl-piperidines				
Pimozide	++	±	±	++
Dibenzoxazepine				
Loxapine	++	++	++	++
Dihydroindolones				
Molindone	+	+	+	++
Butyrophenones				
Haloperidol	+	±	+	+
Droperidol	++	+	+	+
Atypical antipsychotics				
Dibenzodiazepines				
Clozapine	+++	+++	+++	+++
Benzixazoles				
Risperidone	++	++	++	+
Thienobenzo-diazepines				
Olanzapine	++	+	++	++
Dibenzothiazepines				
Quetiapine	++	±	++	++
Imidazolidinones				
Sertindole	++	+	+	+
Substituted benzamides				
Sulpiride	+	±	+	+
Amsulpride	+	±	+	+
Ziprasidone	++	±	+	±

Ratings: ± equivocal; + mild; ++ moderate; +++ strong

dysfunction and abnormal cardiac repolarisation, fulfilling the criteria of autonomic neuropathy.[34] Sustained tachycardia, characterised by an average increase in heart rates by 10 – 15 beats/min, has also been observed in approximately 25% of patients treated with clozapine. This effect is not likely to be a reflex chronotropic response of the heart to hypotension as it has been observed in different positions, and it may pose a serious risk in individuals with compromised left ventricular function. These changes may completely resolve after switching to another antipsychotic agent with less profound blocking effects on muscarinic and adrenergic receptors.[35]

Although unwanted side-effects are less common during therapy with atypical antipsychotics, observational and premarketing clinical randomised studies have also implicated risperidone, quetiapine, and olanzapine in producing clinically relevant hypotension followed by bradycardia.[33,36–41] Thus, in a placebo-controlled, randomised study of 548 patients, intramuscular olanzapine produced a postural decrease in systolic blood pressure twice as often compared with placebo (10.9% vs 4.2%, $P = 0.017$).[40] Treatment with olanzapine was also more often associated with a lower supine diastolic blood pressure (6.3% vs 0.7% patients). In this study, 3% of patients in the olanzapine arm and 1.4% in the placebo arm had a decrease in systolic blood pressure of more than 30 mmHg.[40] Data from 2,300 patients participating in multiple dose-effectiveness trials of quetiapine, whose experience corresponded to approximately 865 patient-years, reported postural hypotension and dizziness related to quetiapine in 7% and 10% patients, respectively.[41]

For a relatively new antipsychotic, ziprasidone, the incidence of postural hypotension was 1.4%, 4.2%, and 4.5% in patients receiving 5 mg, 10 mg, and 20 mg, respectively, of the drug intramuscularly.[42] These changes have been observed for both systolic and diastolic blood pressure. In short-term placebo-controlled trials of oral ziprasidone, the prevalence of orthostatic hypotension as well as dizziness was very low (0.14% and 1.14%, respectively).[43] Of note, haloperidol, clozapine, risperidone, olanzapine, and ziprasidone have also been reported to produce *hypertension* in approximately 1 – 4% of patients.

The assessment of clinical expression of these effects based on the results of *in vitro* binding studies is difficult, as these can merely indicate that a

Table 2. *In Vitro* Receptor Binding Affinity Constants (Ki, nmol/L) of Atypical Antipsychotic Agents

Receptor	Clozapine	Risperidone	Olanzapine	Quetiapine	Sertindole	Ziprasidone
D_1	53	21	10	390	12	9.5
D_2	36	0.44	2.1	69	0.45	2.8
D_4	50	16	28	1600	21	7.4
$5\text{-}HT_{1A}$	710	21	7100	>830	2200	37
$5\text{-}HT_{2A}$	4	0.39	1.9	82	0.20	0.25
$5\text{-}HT_{1C}$	5	6.4	2.8	1500	0.51	0.55
α_1	3.7	0.69	7.3	4.5	1.4	1.9
α_1	51	1.8	140	1100	280	390
H_1	17	88	5.6	21	440	510
M_1	0.98	>5000	2.1	56	260	>10000

The smaller values of Ki indicate the greater receptor affinity.

(Data reproduced with kind permission from ref 45.)

substance binds to a receptor irrespective of its agonistic or antagonistic action (Table 2).[31,44–45] For example, olanzapine exerts a high affinity to muscarinic receptors *in vitro*, but produces mild clinical anticholinergic effects. Similarly, risperidone and ziprasidone have demonstrated a stronger affinity to α_1-adrenoreceptors compared with clozapine.[45] However, the direct effects of α_1-blockade, resulting in orthostatic hypotension, are best known for clozapine. A possible explanation may be the currently limited number of observations with relatively new antipsychotic agents compared with clozapine.

4. Neurocardiogenic syncope
4.1 Pathophysiology of neurocardiogenic syncope
Profound orthostatic hypotension may result in neurocardiogenic syncope (Figure 2). The Committee for Practice Guidelines of the European Society of Cardiology on Management of Syncope[46] defined orthostatic syncope as: 'syncope occurring when the autonomic nervous system is incapacitated resulting in a failure of vasoconstrictor mechanisms and thereby in orthostatic hypotension.' Vasodilatation and bradycardia are characteristic features of neurally-mediated syncope.[47] A reduction in systolic blood pressure and central blood volume caused by upright posture is associated

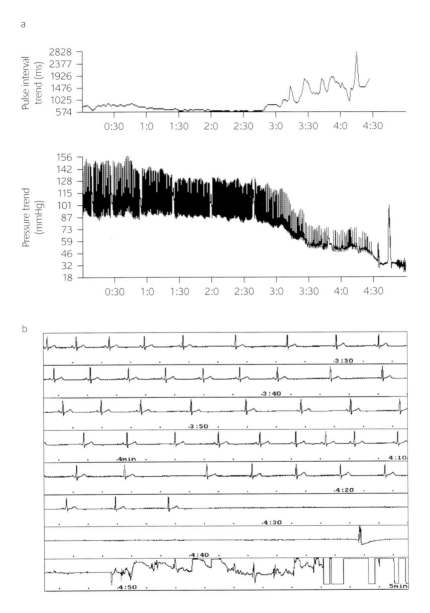

Figure 2. Heart rate and blood pressure trends showing the development of orthostatic hypotension and bradycardia resulting in (a) syncope and (b) an EEG recorded a prolonged period of asystole. Sinus rhythm was restored after a chest blow.

with activation of carotid and aortic baroreceptor reflex, with subsequent increases in circulating catecholamines and cardiac adrenergic tone as an acute response to orthostatic stress. Under these conditions, activation of cardiopulmonary receptors occurs, resulting in increased neural traffic across afferent C fibers leading to central nervous system vasomotor centers. Rostral ventrolateral centers of the medulla respond to this enhanced afferent activity by increasing parasympathetic efferent activity to the heart, leading to reflex bradycardia (cardioinhibitory response), and by decreasing sympathetic outflow, resulting in reflex paradoxical vasodilatation (vasodepressor response) (Figure 3). There is evidence suggesting that in addition to withdrawal of sympathetic tone, alterations in neurohumoral activity is necessary to produce sufficient vasodilatation, resulting in syncope. Epinephrine surge with resultant intense β_2-adrenoreceptor activation further contributes to inappropriate peripheral vasodilatation. The final result is profound hypotension and syncope. This paradoxical reflex is known as a variant of the Bezold-Jarisch reflex. A multiple receptor blockade or agonism by antipsychotic substances at the level of the central nervous system, especially involving $5-HT_{1A}$-serotonergic and GABAergic properties, further contribute to abnormal sympathetic and vagal stimulation.

A decrease in systolic blood pressure to ≥20 mmHg, or a decrease of systolic blood pressure to <90mm Hg during the upright posture, is defined as orthostatic hypotension regardless of the presence or absence of symptoms. In addition, the sedation caused by H_1 histamine receptor blockade, especially during therapy with typical antipsychotics, is associated with the patients remaining in the supine position for extended periods of time which may facilitate venous pooling.

4.2 Antipsychotic treatment and neurocardiogenic syncope

The incidence of this complication varies in different series, from 0.2% with risperidone and olanzapine, 0.6% and 1% with ziprasidone and quetiapine, to 6% with clozapine.[33,38,40–42] Clinical studies in healthy subjects treated with clozapine 25 mg have shown that nearly two thirds experienced orthostatic hypotension, and 47% developed bradycardia below 40 beats/min, with two subjects having sinus arrest with cardiac pauses as

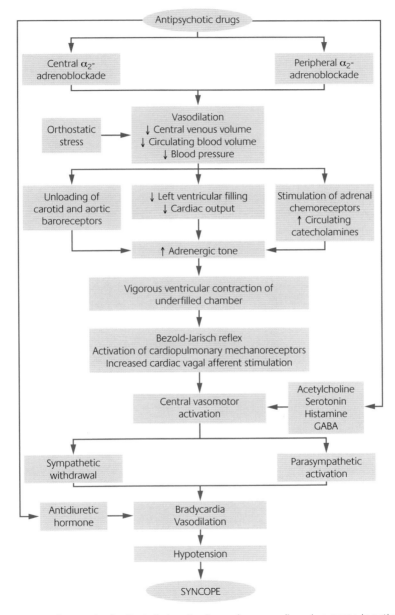

Figure 3. Pathogenesis of orthostatic hypotension and neurocardiogenic syncope in patients treated with antipsychotics drugs.

long as five to seven seconds, and one requiring a chest thump to restore sinus rhythm. Symptomatic bradycardia has been reported in 5% of 41 patients receiving intramuscular injections of ziprasidone 20 mg.[42] In studies of olanzapine, bradycardia was observed in 3.6% of patients after a repeat 5 mg intramuscular injection of olanzapine compared with 1.3% on placebo.[40]

Data from pooled premarketing studies of intramuscular or oral olanzapine have shown that of 850 olanzapine-treated individuals, 64 (7.5%) developed clinically relevant bradycardia, with three cases of sinus arrest lasting up to six seconds that remitted spontaneously.[48] Forty (62.5%) of the 64 cases of bradycardia were associated with a decrement in resting blood pressure or an orthostatic drop, which is consistent with a type of neurally-mediated reflex bradycardia/syncope. Symptoms trended to occur after one hour following intramuscular injection of 5 mg of olanzapine, or after two hours following oral olanzapine 10 mg and persisted for four – six hours. This phenomenon was seen more frequently in normal volunteers without a history of treatment with medications blocking multiple pressor transmitter receptors, non-agitated patients, and patients who had not recently taken antipsychotic medication. Although the ability of antipsychotic agents to block L-type calcium currents in the atria, leading to reduced sinus node automaticity *in vitro*, is pertinent to the clinical observations, these direct effects *in vivo* are probably not sufficient to cause bradycardia and sinus arrest. If sinus node dysfunction occurred, marked bradycardia would be expected rather than the moderate decrements in heart rate in association with hypotension.

It is worth noting that in some studies, (e.g. on clozapine), in which the cause-to-effect relationship between hypotension and syncope was unclear, syncope was regarded as an adverse event related to the central nervous system, whereas hypotension, which occurred in 9% of patients, was attributed to cardiovascular side-effects of the drug. A possible explanation may be that a postural drop in systolic blood pressure may be minimal and may not produce any symptoms, or it may be rather profound and rapidly generates into syncope.

5. Who are predisposed to orthostatic hypotension and syncope?

Orthostatic hypotension, especially if accompanied by syncope, may represent a significant risk in some patients. Apart from lethargy, dizziness, visual disturbances, impaired cognition, and syncope associated with cerebral hypoperfusion, orthostatic hypotension may cause or aggravate myocardial ischemia and renal failure, and may increase risk of falls and bone fractures. Both elderly patients and individuals with pre-existent autonomic disorders or cardiovascular risk factors, such as a history of heart disease, cerebrovascular disorders, hypertension, and diabetes, are particularly sensitive to hypotensive action of antipsychotics and should, therefore, be monitored carefully, especially at the initiation of therapy. The prevalence of this complication in the elderly has been reported to range from 5% to 33%.[49-51] Diminished heart rate response to hypotensive stimuli, impaired α-adrenergic vascular responsiveness, reduced activity of the renin-angiotensin-aldosterone system, decreased plasma vasopressin response to orthostasis, diastolic dysfunction, peripheral neuropathy, and the need for polypharmacy for concurrent comorbidity, which are common in the elderly, are likely to predispose to the development of orthostatic hypotension. As all antipsychotic drugs are metabolised by a hepatic cytochrome system, patients with impaired hepatic function had an approximately 30% lower mean clearance of these substances.

The hypotensive effects may be partially due to individual differences in drug absorption and metabolism. Most antipsychotics are metabolised by the hepatic cytochrome P450 enzymes which demonstrate genetic polymorphism, with about 10% of the population being poor or non-metabolises. For example, approximately 7% of the population in the USA has a genetic deficit in the CYP2D6 cytochrome enzyme that results in a poor metaboliser phenotype.[52] In psychiatric patients phenotyped as deficient in CYP2D6 activity because of significant adverse effects of therapy, 44% of all CYP2D6 gene copies contained alleles associated with inactive CYP2D6 expression.[53] This was more than twice the rate for the occurrence of mutant alleles in patients with little side-effects (21%), and in random subjects from the general population (20%). It has been suggested that screening psychiatric patients for CYP2D6 expression may distinguish metabolic-based therapeutic problems from drug sensitivity caused by other mechanisms. Furthermore, although the CYP3A enzyme is not polymorphic in its distribution among the population, its activity varies over 50-fold in the general population. Consistent with these findings, it has been observed that the normal half-lives of risperidone and its active metabolite, 9-hydroxyreisperidone, are three hours and 17 hours, respectively, but increase to 20 hours and 30 hours in those with little activity of cytochrome CYP2D6 responsible for metabolism of the drug.[37] An example of symptomatic hypotension and bradycardia in a healthy volunteer after ingestion of a single 5 mg dose of olanzapine is presented in Figure 4.[39] The pharmacokinetic studies have linked female gender with a more rapid absorption and a lower clearance of olanzapine, resulting in higher plasma concentrations and a higher likelihood of hypotensive effects of the drug.[54] Indeed, women have been reported to have a greater tendency for the development of orthostatic hypotension with both typical (chlorpromazine, thiriodazine) and atypical drugs (chlorpromazine, risperidone, and olanzapine) compared with men.

6. How to avoid or minimise the risk of orthostatic hypotension and syncope

Although tolerance to the hypotensive effects of antipsychotics occurs in most instances, in some patients orthostatic hypotension may represent a continuing risk. Orthostatic reactions are more likely to persist when drugs are administered intramuscularly, and are more profound with rapid dose escalation. The risk of orthostatic hypotension and syncope may be minimised by limiting the initial dose, e.g. 25 mg twice daily for quetiapine, or 1 mg twice daily for risperidone, in patients without comorbidity, or to 0.5 mg twice daily in the elderly, or in those with renal or hepatic impairment. Since tolerance may develop gradually, the dosage should be titrated upwards over several days until a target dose is reached. If hypotension occurs during titration to the target dose, a return to the previous dose in the titration schedule is appropriate. A permanent dose reduction should be considered if hypotension persists. Data from pooled controlled studies of quetiapine showed that discontinuation of the drug due to refractory hypotension was required in only 0.4% of patients. Antipsychotics known to produce clinically relevant hypotensive reactions should be used with particular caution in patients with established cardiovascular and/or cerebrovascular disease, and in the presence of conditions which would predispose to hypotension, e.g. dehydration, hypovolemia, and concurrent antihypertensive therapy.

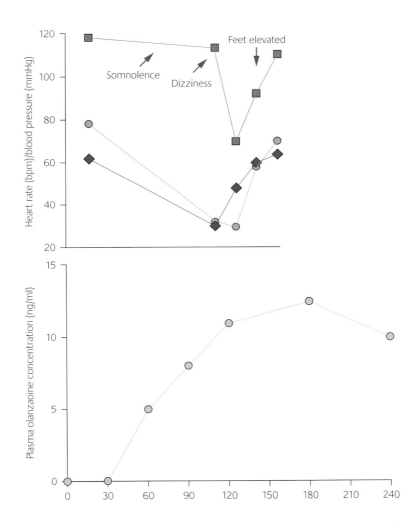

Figure 4. Systolic (purple squares) and diastolic (blue squares) blood pressure, heart rate (green circles), and plasma olanzapine concentrations (yellow circles) in a healthy volunteer after a single 5 mg oral dose of olanzapine, resulting in symptomatic orthostatic hypotension and bradycardia. Please note a rapid increase in plasma olanzapine concentration reaching an unusually high level of 13 ng/ml (typical for olanzapine dosage of 10–15 mg) followed by slow decline.

(Modified from Ref 39. Markowitz JS, De Vane CL, Boulton DW, Liston HL, Risch SC. Hypotension and bradycardia in a healthy volunteer following a single 5 mg dose of olanzapine. *J Clin Pharmacol* 42 pp. 104–106, copyright © 2002 by Sage Publications, Inc. Reprinted by permission of Sage Publications Inc.)

Patients should be advised to avoid abrupt postural changes, standing still for a prolonged period of time, prolonged recumbence during the day-time, straining during micturition and defecation, hyperventilation, severe exertion, large meals with a high content of refined carbohydrates, and alcohol. Some patients may benefit from support stockings, volume expansion by fluid intake of 2 – 2.5 L/day, or agents with sympathetic vasoconstrictor properties which increase peripheral resistance and reduce the tendency for gravitational downward displacement of central volume, such as pure α-adrenergic agents, norepinephrine and metaraminol. Midodrine may be effective in protecting the patients with impaired baroreflex activity from accidental orthostatic hypotension due to its competing action with antipsychotics at α_1-adrenoreceptors and subsequent restoration of reflex vasoconstriction.[55] Additional benefit may be attained with salt retaining steroids (fludrocortisone). However, the use of epinephrine may paradoxically worsen antipsychotic-induced hypotension by virtue of β-adrenergic stimulation in the presence of α-blockade and is thus contraindicated.

7. Effects of antipsychotic drugs on heart rate variability

In light of the evidence of the association of antipsychotic drug therapy and sudden cardiac death, a number of studies have investigated the effects of antipsychotics on heart rate variability as the measure of autonomic cardiovascular status.[56–58] The first indirect implication of antipsychotic agents in impaired heart rate variability was based on the observation of an absence of changes in heart rate with respiration, and the absence of changes in heart rate and blood pressure after valsalva maneuver, hand grip, cold-pressor, or mental stress testing, accompanied by a significant reduction of plasma norepinephrine levels and normal epinephrine levels, suggesting vagal withdrawal and an increase in sympathetic activity.[59] Of note, a positive pressor effect of tyramine indicated that such autonomic dysfunction was likely to be central in origin.

Clozapine, the most extensively investigated agent, has been proven to significantly increase the low-frequency component of total spectrum power which reflects enhanced sympathetic stimulation, and to decrease the high-frequency component which reflects parasympathetic activity.[58] These effects can be accounted for by the anticholinergic and antihistaminergic properties of clozapine.[60] Haloperidol, sertindole, and olanzapine have been reported to produce less pronounced effects on heart rate variability which is mediated mainly by an increase in sympathetic tone. As these agents have no significant blocking effect on β-adrenoreceptors, an indirect sympathetic activation via α-receptor blocking activity is likely to be the underlying mechanism. Figure 5 shows significantly reduced heart rate variability during therapy with clozapine compared with olanzapine.[57]

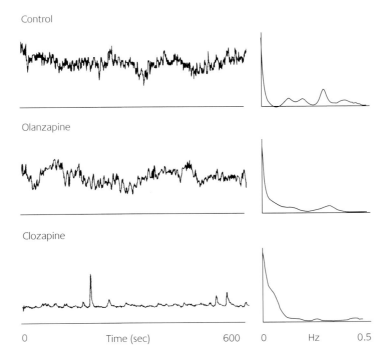

Figure 5. Tachograms (left) and power spectral analysis of heart rate variability in a healthy subject and patients receiving olanzapine and clozapine. The power spectra show heart rate variability in all frequency bands (y-axis, ms 2/103 Hz).

(Modified with permission from Ref 57. Cohen H, Loewenthal U, Matar M, Kotler M. Association of autonomic dysfunction and clozapine. *Br J Psychiatry* 2001; 179: 167–171.)

8. Conclusions

Antipsychotic drugs represent a pharmacologically and structurally diverse group of agents with the main therapeutic action being realised through the blockade of dopamine receptors (typical antipsychotics), or serotonin-dopamine antagonism (atypical antipsychotics) in the central nervous system. However, both typical and atypical antipsychotic drugs exhibit high affinity for other numerous receptors, including histaminergic, α- and β-adrenergic, muscarinic, and GABAergic, which inevitably results in various unwanted effects on other systems. Orthostatic hypotension is the most common cardiovascular adverse effect of antipsychotic treatment which occurs in a substantial proportion of patients, even at therapeutic levels. Profound hypotension and neurally-mediated syncope are particularly sinister complications as they may result in cardiorespiratory arrest and sudden death. Although contemporary experimental and clinical data have provided a significantly better understanding of the role of different receptors in central cardiovascular regulation, the complex interplay between multiple receptor subtypes and their action at different levels of the central nervous system to elicit changes induced by receptor agonists and antagonists, remain an area of further investigation. To date, pharmacologic and clinical evidence is not sufficient to clearly rank existing antipsychotic drugs with respect to their adverse cardiovascular effects.[61] Antipsychotic agents with a lower incidence of side-effects and better risk/benefit ratio have been developed, such as ziprasidone, iloperidone, and aripiprazole, which do not block adrenergic, muscarinic, and histaminergic receptors to an appreciable extent and have, therefore, a low liability for side-effects typically associated with poor patient compliance.

References

1. Ruchena D, Mullen PE, Burgess P, et al. Sudden death in psychiatric patients. Br J Psychiatry 1998; **172**: 331–336.

2. Appleby L, Thomas S, Ferrier N, et al. Sudden unexplained death in psychiatric in-patients. Br J Psychiatry 2000; **176**: 405–406.

3. Martin R, Cloningerv C, Guze S, et al. Mortality in a follow-up of 500 psychiatric outpatients II: Case-specific mortality. Arch Gen Psychiatry 1985; **42**: 58–66.

4. Chute D, Grove C, Rajasekhara B, et al. Schizophrenia and sudden death: a medical examiner case study. Am J For Med Path 1999; **20**: 131–135.

5. Jusic N, Lader M. Postmortem antipsychotic drug concentrations and unexplained deaths. Br J Psychiatry 1994; **165**: 787–791.

6. Reilly JG, Ayis SA, Ferrier IN, et al. Thioridazine and sudden unexplained death in psychiatric in-patients. Br J Psychiatry 2002; **180**: 515–522.

7. Glassman AH, Bigger JT, Jr. Antipsychotic drugs: prolonged QTc interval, *torsades de pointes*, and sudden death. *Am J Psychiatry* 2001; **158**: 1774–1782.

8. Welsh R, Chue P. Antipsychotic agents and QT changes. *J Psychiatry Neurosci* 2000; **25**: 154–160.

9. Buckley NA, Sanders P. Cardiovascular effects of antipsychotic drugs. *Drug Saf* 2000; **23**: 215–228.

10. Autonomic Failure: A Textbook of Clinical Disorders of the Autonomic Nervous System, 4th ed. (Mathias CJ, Bannister R, ed). New York: Oxford University Press Inc., 1999: pp37 – 62.

11. Bonner TI, Buckley NJ, Young AC, Brann MR. Identification of a family of muscarinic acetylcholine receptor genes. *Science* 1987; **237**: 527–532.

12. Hulme EC, Birdsall NJM, Buckley NJ. Muscarinic receptor subtypes. *Annu Rev Pharmacol Toxicol* 1990; **30**: 633–673.

13. Meyer EC, Sommers DK. Possible mechanisms of anticholinergic drug-induced bradycardia. *Eur J Clin Pharmacol* 1988; **35**: 503–506.

14. Saito K, Yoshioka M, Kohya T, *et al.* Involvement of muscarinic M_1 receptor in the central pathway of the serotonin-induced Bezold-Jarisch reflex in rats. *J Auton Nerv Syst* 1994; **49**: 61–68.

15. Taira CA, Enero MA. Central α_1- and α_2-adrenoreceptors and brain cholinergic stimulation in sinoaortic denervated rats. *Eur J Pharmacol* 1994; **271**: 9–16.

16. Robinson SE. Serotonin-cholinergic interactions in blood pressure control in the rat. *Fed Proc* 1984; **43**: 21–24.

17. McCall RB, Patel BN, Harris L. Effects of serotonin1 and serotonin2 receptors in the central regulation of the cardiovascular system. *Pharmacol Rev* 1994; **46**: 231–243.

18. Ramage A. Central cardiovascular regulation and 5-hydroxytryptamine receptors. *Brain Res Bull* 2001; **56**: 425–439.

19. Knowles ID, Ramage AG. Evidence for a role for central 5HT2B as well as 5-HT_{2A} receptors in cardiovascular regulation in anaesthetized rats. *Br J Pharmacol* 1999; **128**: 530–542.

20. Pires JG, Silva SR, Ramage AG, *et al.* Evidence that 5-HT_3 receptors in the nucleus tractus solitarius and other brainstem areas modulate the vagal bradycardia evoked by activation of the von Bezold-Jarisch reflex in the anesthetized rat. *Brain Res* 1998; **791**: 229–234.

21. Sevoz C, Nosjean A, Callera JC, *et al.* Stimulation of 5-HT_3 receptors in the NTS inhibits the cardiac Bezold-Jarisch reflex response. *Am J Physiol* 1996; **271**: H80–H87.

22. Gallacher M, Ramage AG. Evidence which indicates that the activation of central 5-HT_{1Da} receptors can cause hypotension in anesthetized rats. *Br J Pharmacol* 1006; **117**: 142P.

23. Kosinski D, Grubb BP, Temesy-Annos P. The use of serotonin reuptake inhibitors in the treatment of neurally mediated cardiovascular disorders. *J Serotonin Res* 1994; **1**: 85–90.

24. Bago M, Dean C. Sympathoinhibition from ventrolateral periaqueductal gray mediated by 5-HT(1A) receptors in the RVLM. *Am J Physiol Regul Integr Comp Physiol* 2001; **280**: R976–R984.

25. Tangri KK, Gupta GP, Vrat S. Role of histamine receptor in mesencephalic nucleus dorsalis raphe in cardiovascular regulation. *Naunyn Schmiedebergs Arch Pharmacol* 1989; **339**: 557–563.

26. Granata AR, Reis DJ. Hypotension and bradycardia elicited by histamine into the C1 area of the rostral ventrolateral medulla. *Eur J Pharmacol* 1987; **136**: 157–162.

27. Spyer KM. Central nervous mechanisms contributing to cardiovascular control. *J Physiol* 1994; **474**: 1–19.

28. McLeod RL, Gertner SB, Hey JA. Hemodynamic profile of activation of histamine H_3 receptors by R-alpha-methylhistamine in the guinea pig. *Gen Pharmacol* 1996; **27**: 1001–1007.

29. Kajekar R, Chen CY, Mutoh T, *et al.* GABA(A) receptor activation at medullary sympathetic neurons contributes to post exercise hypotension. *Am J Physiol Heart Circ Physiol* 2002; **282**: H1615–H1624.

30. Li YW, Guyenet PG. Neuronal inhibition by a $GABA_B$ receptor agonist in the rostral ventrolateral medulla of the rat. *Am J Physiol* 1995; **268**: R428–R437.

31. Stanniland C, Taylor D. Tolerability of atypical antipsychotics. *Drug Saf* 2000; **22**: 195–214.

32. Silver H, Kogan H, Zlotogorski D. Postural hypotension in chronically medicated schizophrenics. *J Clin Psychiatry* 1990; **51**: 459–462.

33. Clozaril® (clozapine) tablets prescribing information April 2001, pp1–22. http://www.fda.gov/

34. Pretorius JL, Phillips M, Langley RW, *et al.* Comparison of clozapine and haloperidol on some autonomic and psychomotor functions, and on serum prolactin concentration, in healthy subjects. *J Clin Pharmacol* 2001; **52**: 322–326.

35. Cohen H, Loweenthal U, Matar M, *et al.* Reversal of pathologic cardiac parameters after transition from clozapine to olanzapine treatment: A case report. *Clin Neuropharm* 2001; **2**: 106–108.

36. Himstreet JE, Daya M. Hypotension and orthostasis following a risperidone overdose. *Ann Pharmacother* 1998; **32**: 267.

37. Product information. Risperdal (risperidone). Titusville, NJ: Janssen Pharmaceuticals, Inc., 1993.

38. Risperdal® (risperidone). Revision 2 June 1999, pp1 – 3. http://www.fda.gov/

39. Markowitz JS, DeVane CL, Boulton DW, *et al.* Hypotension and bradycardia in a healthy volunteer following a single 5 mg dose of olanzapine. *J Clin Pharmacol* 2002; **42**: 104–106.

40. FDA Psychopharmacological Drugs Advisory Committee Briefing Document for ZYPREXA® IntraMuscular (olanzapine for injection), 11 January 2001, pp1–115. http://www.fda.gov/

41. Seroquel® (quetiapine fumarate) tablets. Revision January 2001, pp1–25. http://www.fda.gov/

42. FDA Psychopharmacological Drugs Advisory Committee Briefing Document for Ziprasidone Mesylate for Intramuscular Injection, 15 February 2001, pp1–75. http://www.fda.gov/

43. FDA Psychopharmacological Drugs Advisory Committee Briefing Document for Zeldox® (Ziprasidone-HCl), 14 June 2000, pp1–173. http://www.fda.gov/

44. Casey DE. Side effect profiles of new antipsychotic agents. *J Clin Psychiatry* 1997; **58** (Suppl 10): 55–62.

45. Markowitz JS, Brown CS, Moore TR. Atypical antipsychotics. Part I: Pharmacology, pharmacokinetics, and efficacy. *Ann Pharmacother* 1999; **33**: 73–85.

46. Brignole M, Alboni P, Benditt D, *et al.* Task Force on Syncope, European Society of Cardiology. Guidelines on management (diagnosis and treatment) of syncope. *Eur Heart J* 2001; **22**: 1256–1306.

47. Benditt DG. Neurally mediated syncopal syndromes: Pathophysiological concepts and clinical evaluation. *Pacing Clin Electrophysiol* 1997; **20**: 572–584.

48. FDA Psychopharmacological Drugs Advisory Committee. Addendum to Briefing Document for ZYPREXA® IntraMuscular (olanzapine for injection), 19 January 2001, pp1–49. http://www.fda.gov/

49. Mcmanus DQ, Arvantis LA, Kowalcyk BB. Quetiapine, a novel antipsychotic: experience in elderly patients with psychotic disorders: Seroquel Trial; 48 Study Group. *J Clin Psychiatry* 1999; **60**: 292–298.

50. Tariot PN, Salzman Yeung PP, *et al.* Long-term use of quetiapine in elderly patients with psychotic disorders. *Clin Ther* 2000; **22**: 1068–1684.

51. Verhaeverbeke I, Mets T. Drug-induced orthostatic hypotension in the elderly: avoiding its onset. *Drug Saf* 1997; **17**: 105–118.

52. Steimer W, Mueller B, Leucht S, *et al.* Prevalence of cytochrome P450 2D6 (CYP2D6) and serotonin transporter (5HTT) polymorphisms in depressed inpatients compared to a control group. *Clin Chem* 2000; **46**: A210 (Abstract).

53. Chen S, Chou WH, Blouin RA, *et al.* The cytochrome P450 2D6 (CYP2D6) enzyme polymorphism: Screening costs and influence on clinical outcomes in psychiatry. *Clin Pharmacol Ther* 1996; **60**: 522–534.

54. Kelly DL, Conley RR, Tamminga CA. Differential olanzapine plasma concentrations by sex in a fixed-dose study. *Schizophr Res* 1999; **40**: 101–104.

55. Kurihara J, Takata Y, Sizuki S, *et al.* Effect of midodrine on chlorpromazine orthostatic hypotension in rabbits: Comparison with amezinium, etilefrine and droxidopa. *Biol Pharm Bull* 2000; **23**: 1445–1449.

56. Rechlin T. The effects of psychopharmacological therapy on heart rate variation *Nervenarzt* 1995; **66**: 678–685 [Abstract].

57. Cohen H, Loweenthal U, Matar M, *et al.* Association of autonomic dysfunction and clozapine: heart rate variability and risk for sudden death in patients with schizophrenia on long-term psychotropic medication. *Br J Psychiatry* 2001; **179**: 167–171.

58. Agelink MW, Majewski T, Wurthmann C, *et al.* Effects of newer atypical antipsychotics on autonomic neurocardiac function: A comparison between amisulpride, olanzapine, sertindole, and clozapine. *J Clin Psychopharmacol* 2001; **21**: 8–1113.

59. Karet FE, Dickerson JE, Brown J, *et al.* Bovril
and moclobemide: A novel therapeutic
strategy for central autonomic failure.
Lancet 1994; **344**: 1263–1265.
60. Zann TP, Pickar D. Autonomic effects of
clozapine in schizophrenia: Comparison
with placebo and fluphenazine. *Biol
Psychiatry* 1993; **34**: 3–12.
61. Casey DE. Barriers to progress – the
impact of tolerability problems. *Int Clin
Psychopharmacol* 2001; **16(Suppl 1)**:
S15–S19.

Heart muscle disease and antipsychotic therapy

Andrew A. Grace

Department of Cardiology, Papworth Hospital, Cambridge CB3 8RE
and University of Cambridge, Section of Cardiovascular Biology, Department of
Biochemistry, Tennis Court Road, Cambridge CB2 1QW, United Kingdom

Correspondence: Andrew A. Grace Ph.D. F.R.C.P. Section of Cardiovascular Biology,
Department of Biochemistry, University of Cambridge,
Tennis Court Road, Cambridge CB2 1QW
Telephone: +44 (0)1480 364 350 (Secretary)
Fax: +44 (0)1223 333 345
Email: ag@mole.bio.cam.ac.uk

1. Introduction

An increased risk of sudden death in patients with major psychoses is well documented.[1–2] Unnatural deaths clearly contribute substantially,[1–3] but the incidence of natural sudden cardiac deaths is also increased.[2–4] These deaths occur against the background of the poor physical health of these patients,[5] with cardiovascular risk aggravated by heavy cigarette consumption and obesity.[5] Although the data is not complete, a high incidence of coronary artery disease and hypertension[6] almost certainly increases the likelihood of heart muscle disease in these patients presenting most usually as chronic heart failure. The presence of heart disease in any population can complicate the use of therapeutic drugs, particularly if these drugs are known to both bind to, and influence, the activity of cardiac ion channels,[7] as is the case with many of the currently used antipsychotic agents.[8]

This chapter has two main purposes: (i) to examine the extent to which intrinsic heart muscle disease provides a risk for sudden death in patients given antipsychotic agents; and, (ii) to present the data implicating antipsychotic agents as a direct cause of myocarditis and cardiomyopathy. These relatively rare, devastating but potentially reversible complications should be considered in day-to-day practice by medical professionals.

2. Risk is enhanced in patients with heart muscle disease

Sudden cardiac death is the single most common cause of death,[9-11] responsible for an annual toll estimated at 70,000 deaths in the UK[12] and 300,000 deaths in the USA.[10-11] Ventricular arrhythmias are responsible for sudden cardiac death and are due to disturbances of the normal heartbeat,[9] often arising from scar tissue in the ventricular myocardium, although the trigger may be ischemic in the setting of coronary disease.[11]

Ventricular arrhythmias occur in several clinical settings. Congenital long-QT syndromes, for example, are uncommon, usually affect young people, and predispose to *torsades de pointes*, a ventricular arrhythmia relatively specific to this condition.[13-14] However, most ventricular arrhythmias occur in older patients with heart muscle disease, with a clinical syndrome referred to as chronic heart failure that has resulted from previous myocardial infarction or from cardiomyopathy.[10-11] Improvements in the treatment of acute myocardial infarction have resulted in improved survival, and as a result the incidence of chronic heart failure has increased and is considered by some to have reached epidemic proportions.[15] Chronic heart failure is a major cause of morbidity and mortality, with approximately half of the affected patients dying suddenly from ventricular arrhythmias.[10-11]

The normal function of the heart results from the combined activities of ion channels responsible for action potentials and excitation-contraction coupling. Repolarisation of cardiac action potentials is mediated by outward currents passing predominantly through potassium channels.[16-17] The mechanistic link that substantially accounts for the enhanced risk with certain drugs,[17] both in the functional long-QT syndromes and in structural heart muscle disease, is a reduction in net potassium channel function leading in turn to delayed action potential repolarisation.[13,16] Accordingly, in most patients with congenital long-QT syndrome loss-of-function mutations in cardiac potassium channel genes (e.g. mutations in *KCNQ1* causing LQT1, or mutations in *KCNH2 (HERG)* causing LQT2) lead to delayed repolarisation, manifested by QT prolongation on the surface electrocardiogram.[13-14] The mechanisms that then link QT prolongation to *torsades de pointes* and, thereby, to syncope and sudden cardiac death are not resolved, but are the subject of intensive research. By contrast, in heart muscle disease, whilst mutations in potassium channel genes are not seen the numbers of potassium channels are reduced.[16-18] The final net electrophysiological effect in heart muscle disease is therefore the same as in the long QT syndromes, i.e. delayed repolarisation (Figure 1). Delayed repolarisation taken together with other transcriptionally-mediated electrophysiological and structural changes, including cellular hypertrophy, leads to a potent substrate for ventricular arrhythmias, and the risk of sudden cardiac death.[16,11] Super-imposed drug-associated inhibition of potassium channel function in both settings can be catastrophic.

3. Drugs enhance risk in heart muscle disease

The number of drugs implicated in acquired long QT syndrome and *torsades de pointes* has increased enormously.[8,17] When such drugs are given to patients with heart disease, the risk of ventricular arrhythmias is enhanced and is a serious issue that needs to be kept in mind, both generally when using these drugs and specifically in these patients.[8] Against this background, one of the hurdles to be surmounted before a new drug receives approval for market release is to establish its likely cardiac risk profile.[9] Almost all the drugs so far identified with these characteristics selectively inhibit the rapid component of the delayed rectifier potassium current (I_{Kr})[7] that is encoded by the *KCNH2* gene also known as HERG.

The best evidence for drug-induced risk in those with heart disease *per se* mostly comes from the study of antiarrhythmic agents that inhibit I_{Kr}.[19-20] As an example, in the Stroke Prevention in Atrial Fibrillation (SPAF) trial when patients with chronic heart failure were given such drugs they had a relative

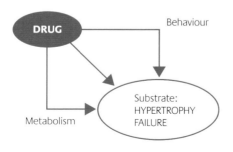

Figure 1. General principles of how drugs modified by behaviour and metabolism act on the substrate of the diseased myocardium to generate arrhythmia risk.

risk of cardiac death of 4.7 compared with those without such a history.[21] The problem in the interpretation of these data was that the patients who received antiarrhythmic agents had more severe heart disease and a higher predicted risk anyway.[21–22] These sorts of issues are a recurring theme and appear to confound simple interpretations that support the suggestion that I_{Kr} block enhances risk in chronic heart failure. For example, in trials conducted in this setting to assess the use of class III antiarrhythmic agents that selectively inhibit I_{Kr},[19–20] d-sotalol enhanced risk[19,23] whereas no effect on mortality was seen with dofetilide.[20] The explanation for the different outcomes may lie in trial design,[20] but the dofetilide data also suggest that excess risk may not be a necessary outcome of I_{Kr} blockade.

No matter how the individual data are interpreted the evidence taken together is sufficiently strong to force consideration of the risks of underlying heart disease in drug prescribing. Accordingly, a major challenge for healthcare professionals is to identify patients with heart disease prior to antipsychotic drug prescription so as to minimise iatrogenic risks.[8] Illustrating the potential difficulties are the occasional sporadic reports of therapeutic drugs causing sudden cardiac death in individuals with no known heart disease. In one recent example, a 22-year-old American student with absolutely no relevant past history was leading a teenage exchange group in West Africa.[24] He developed symptoms interpreted as being due to malaria and was given the antimalarial, halofantrine. Shortly thereafter he fell to the ground dead and was found at post-mortem examination to have hypertrophic cardiomyopathy. Several similar, albeit less graphic, accounts also feature in the psychiatric literature.[25–26]

4. Evidence that antipsychotic drugs enhance risk in heart muscle disease

Patients with major psychiatric disease have a higher incidence of coronary artery disease[5–6] and hypertension.[6] These disorders are both major risks for the development of heart muscle disease.[11,15] The epidemiological data on the incidence and prevalence of chronic heart failure in any population is more difficult to obtain,[15] and in patients with psychoses there are no data. This is at least partially explained by the relative lack of interest in the physical well-being of these patients.[5,27] These factors conspire to limit data directly implicating antipsychotic agents in risk in patients with heart disease. For example, there are no studies that have examined the incidence of ambulant ventricular arrhythmias in patients with heart disease given antipsychotic drug treatment.[28] Interestingly, in those without cardiac disease given these drugs the risk of ambulant arrhythmia is apparently not increased.[29]

The limited data available strongly imply that heart disease does increase the risks of using antipsychotic drugs. For example, an autopsy-based survey from Finland was one of the first to highlight the potential risks for sudden cardiac death inherent to antipsychotic or antidepressant agents.[30] The report documented 49 cases of sudden cardiac death in patients mostly receiving either thioridazine or phenothiazines, and in over half of these patients cardiac or coronary abnormalities were found at post-mortem examination.[30] Cardiac hypertrophy was observed in 11 cases and cellular fibrosis was also commonly observed, which at the time was attributed possibly to phenothiazines. Similarly, the Tennessee Medicaid study is a retrospective cohort study of half a million persons in the USA with a 2.5 year follow-up.[31–32] In this study there were 1,487 cases of sudden cardiac death (11.6 events per 10,000 person-years of observation). The relative risk of sudden death for individuals receiving antipsychotic drugs was 2.39 greater than for non-users of antipsychotics (Figure 2). Although there were several problems based mainly on the retrospective nature of the analyses, the study documented directly for the first time the importance of the presence of heart disease as a risk factor for sudden cardiac death in patients given antipsychotic drugs. The classifications of heart disease were very broad, but nevertheless categorised risk sharply in those patients given antipsychotics between those individuals with no heart disease (relative risk, RR = 1.60), versus mild, moderate, or severe heart disease (RR = 3.18, 2.12, and 3.53, respectively). The need for further prospective evaluations has been noted.[32]

Thioridazine has potent potassium channel blocking activity[33] and is a well-documented cause of the acquired long QT syndrome[34] and *torsades de pointes*, and is particularly lethal when taken in overdose.[35] These observations have led to severe restrictions being imposed on its use.[8] In the UK, the Committee on the Safety of Medicines (CSM) has restricted the drug to second-line use in patients with schizophrenia, and it requires careful cardiological evaluation before it is prescribed. Concerns regarding the use of

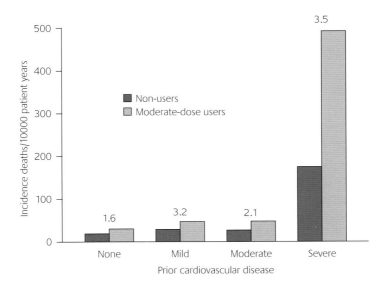

Figure 2. The Tennessee Medicaid study.[31] Rates of sudden cardiac death in current users of moderate dose antipsychotics (thioridazine >100 mg/day or its equivalent) and non-users, by severity of cardiovascular disease. Rates of death in non-users are standardised to the age and sex distribution of the cohort. P values test the difference between moderate dose current users and non-users.

thioridazine in patients with known heart disease is further supported by more recent data from a study designed to examine the risks for sudden death in those with major psychiatric disease from the North of England.[36] Thioridazine was the only antipsychotic drug identified as an independent risk factor for sudden death. The two other major risks were the presence of coronary artery disease (odds ratio = 17.0), and hypertension (odds ratio = 13.6). Unfortunately, the study was not sufficiently powered to determine the extent to which heart disease and thioridazine were synergistic in respect of risk.[36–37]

5. Using antipsychotic drugs in patients with heart disease

Amongst the most important identifiable risk factors to consider when initiating antipsychotic drugs are the presence of heart disease, including heart failure and a history of arrhythmias or myocardial infarction,[6,8] and appropriate clinical measures to identify these risks should be taken. One serious problem is that psychiatrists and family physicians are generally quite poor at recognising physical conditions in psychiatric patients.[1,5] This may be improved by using structured physical assessments that have been shown to be effective at revealing physical illness in this population.[38-39] A barrier to specific investigations is the fact that prescribers are not usually familiar with electrocardiographic interpretation. However, the apparent risk of ventricular arrhythmias with the newer antipsychotic agents is low, and routine pre-treatment ECGs to look for evidence of heart disease or for QT prolongation are thought by most commentators to be unnecessary.[40] In some patients, for example, elderly patients and those with heart disease, a routine ECG may be worthwhile.[40]

Although thioridazine has been clearly associated with risk, it should be assumed for the time being that all antipsychotic agents may have this potential,[37] an idea supported by numerous isolated reports.[25-26] Indeed some reports have recommended that the newer antipsychotics are generally best avoided in patients with serious heart disease.[37,40-41] One of the main problems with the currently available data is that clinical trials have generally excluded complicated patients – including those with heart disease – so for general guidance one has to look elsewhere. The largest relevant experience of patients with heart disease has been gained with antiarrhythmic drugs.[22,42-43] For some of the antiarrhythmic drugs, the use of which are frequently complicated by ventricular arrhythmias, their initiation in hospital with ECG monitoring has been suggested[22,42-43] but this is not usually practical for prescription of antipsychotic agents.

It is possible that the risks of using newer antipsychotic agents in heart disease patients will be clinically acceptable but trials will be needed. In this regard, recent studies of the use of antidepressant medication following acute myocardial infarction provide a model of how such trials could be designed,[44-45] and have been encouraging despite earlier concerns.[46] Specifically, in the Sertraline Antidepressant Heart Attack Trial (SADHART)[44] the selective serotonin re-uptake inhibitor, sertraline, has been shown to be both safe and effective in patients with depression and impaired heart function.[44] This type of painstaking clinical investigation highlights the need for further prospective studies of the risks of antipsychotic treatment.[45]

6. Evidence that antipsychotic therapy causes heart muscle disease

Clozapine remains one of the most effective agents for the treatment of refractory schizophrenia.[47–50] The first isolated case reports of myocarditis[51–52] and cardiomyopathy[53] associated with clozapine seemed relatively insignificant initially when compared with those for adverse haematological reactions. However, the evidence that clozapine can cause myocarditis and cardiomyopathy is now persuasive,[54–55] with data gathering facilitated by the availability of databases such as the Clozaril National Registry in the USA[56] that were set up to protect patients against haematological risks.[54–55] The first systematic investigation of the extent and characteristics of the heart muscle disease due to clozapine was based on reports made to the Australian Adverse Drug Reaction Committee (ADRAC).[54] Between January 1993 and March 1999, 8,000 Australian patients received clozapine, with myocarditis occurring in 15 cases including five deaths (1000–2000 fold increase over that predicted), and dilated cardiomyopathy in eight cases (a five-fold increase). The subsequent report based on data available to the Food and Drug Administration (FDA) showed a similar picture: between September 1989 and December 1999, 189,405 individuals in the USA received clozapine with 28 reports of myocarditis (321 fatal cases per million patient years), and 41 cases of dilated cardiomyopathy (five-fold increase)[55] (Table 1). The post-marketing surveillance by the manufacturers, Novartis, further supported this general level of risk.[57–58]

Although relatively rare, the clinical picture is poor for patients presenting with drug-associated myocarditis,[54–55,59–60] and to achieve a successful outcome a high level of clinical monitoring is needed. In a letter to health care providers in the United States in April 2002, Novartis, the manufacturer of the drug cautioned:

"...the possibility of myocarditis should be considered in patients receiving clozapine who present with unexplained fatigue, dyspnoea, tachypnoea, fever, chest pains, palpitations, other signs or symptoms of heart failure, or electrocardiographic findings such as ST-T wave abnormalities or

Table 1. Clozapine-induced heart disease in the USA.[56]

Variable	Cardiomyopathy	Myocarditits
Total number	41	28
Number confirmed	22	17
Age	20–59	25–66
Sex (male)	32	15
Treatment duration	2 wk – 7 yr	2 wk – 7 yr
Deaths	10 (24)	18 (64)

(La Grenade L, Graham D, Trontell A. Myocarditis and cardiomyopathy associated with clozapine use in the United States. *N Engl J Med*, 345; 3: 224. Copyright © 2001 Massachusetts Medical Society. All rights reserved.)

arrhythmias. It is not known whether eosinophilia is a reliable predictor for myocarditis. Tachycardia which has been associated with clozapine treatment has also been noted as a presenting sign in patients with myocarditis. Therefore, tachycardia during the first month of therapy warrants close monitoring for other signs of myocarditis. The prompt discontinuation of clozapine is warranted upon suspicion of myocarditis."

This advice should be followed in all patients started on this drug. The mechanisms whereby clozapine damages the heart are unknown but the clinical picture fits most easily with a hypersensitivity myocarditis as previously reported with other drug associations[59–60] and associated with eosinophilic infiltration of the myocardium (Figure 3). Suggestions of specific triggers factors, such as genetic predisposition, modified metabolism and

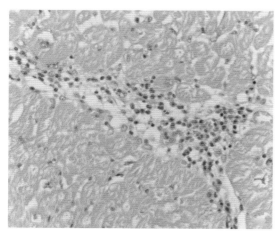

Figure 3. Section of myocardium showing the effects of hypersensitivity myocarditis with diffuse infiltration with eosinophils (Haematoxylin and Eosin x 250). Other features include myocytolysis and necrosis.

Table 2. Antipsychotic drugs for which two or more reports of cardiomyopathy have been registered with the WHO database.[63]

Drug	Cases	Total reports	Information component −2SD
Clozapine	213	24,730	3.14
Other antipsychotic	89	60,775	0.40
Lithium	17	6,315	0.76
Cholrporomazine	14	5,386	0.63
Fluphenazine	8	2,242	0.62

(*BMJ* 2001; 322: 1207–1209, with permission from the BMJ Publishing Group.)

altered environmental conditions, most specifically high ozone[61] have not been substantiated.

Although clozapine is the antipsychotic drug most fully documented as a cause of cardiac muscle disease there is also evidence that other antipsychotic drugs can cause a similar syndrome, e.g. quetiapine.[62] In addition, a pharmacovigilance data mining approach, the Bayesian Confidence Propagation network of the World Health Organisation (WHO) adverse drug reaction database, suggested an enhanced risk with lithium, chlorpromazine, fluphenazine, haloperidol, and risperidone[63] (Table 2) , and all of these agents need further investigation.

References

1. Felker B, Yazel JJ, Short D. Mortality and medical comorbidity among psychiatric patients: A review. *Psychiatr Serv* 1996; **47**: 1356–1363.
2. Appleby L, Thomas S, Ferrier N, *et al.* Sudden unexplained death in psychiatric in-patients. *Br J Psychiatry* 2000; **176**: 405–406.
3. Brown S, Inskip H, Barraclough B. Causes of the excess mortality of schizophrenia. *Br J Psychiatry* 2000; **177**: 212–217.
4. Ebert MH, Shader RI. Cardiovascular effects. In: *Psychotropic Drug Side Effects: Clinical and theoretical perspectives* (Shader RI, DiMascio A, ed.). Baltimore: Williams and Wilkins. 1970; pp:149–163.
5. Phelan M, Stradins L, Morrison S. Physical health of people with severe mental illness. *BMJ* 2001; **322**: 443–444.
6. Buckley NA, Sanders P. Cardiovascular adverse effects of antipsychotic drugs. *Drug Saf* 2000; **23**: 215–228.
7. Yang T, Snyders D, Roden DM. Drug block of I(kr): Model systems and relevance to human arrhythmias. *J Cardiovasc Pharmacol* 2001; **38**: 737–744.
8. Glassman AH, Bigger JT, Jr. Antipsychotic drugs: Prolonged QTc interval, *torsades de pointes*, and sudden death. *Am J Psychiatry* 2001; **158**: 1774–1782.
9. Noble D. Unraveling the genetics and mechanisms of cardiac arrhythmia. *Proc Natl Acad Sci U S A* 2002; **99**: 5755–5756.
10. Zipes DP, Wellens HJJ. Sudden cardiac death. *Circulation* 1998; **98**: 2334–2351.
11. Huikuri HV, Castellanos A, Myerburg RJ. Sudden death due to cardiac arrhythmias. *N Engl J Med* 2001; **345**: 1473–1482.
12. British Pacing and Electrophysiology Group Committee. Submission to National Institute for Clinical Excellence. May 2000.
13. Keating MT, Sanguinetti MC. Molecular and cellular mechanisms of cardiac arrhythmias. *Cell* 2001; **104**: 569–580.

14. Schwartz PJ, Priori SG, Spazzolini C, *et al*. Genotype-phenotype correlation in the long-QT syndrome: Gene-specific triggers for life-threatening arrhythmias. *Circulation* 2001; **103**: 89–95.

15. Redfield MM. Heart Failure – An epidemic of uncertain proportions. *N Engl J Med* 2002; **347**: 1442–1444.

16. Tomaselli GF, Marban E. Electrophysiological remodeling in hypertrophy and heart failure. *Cardiovasc Res* 1999; **42**: 270–283.

17. Haverkamp W, Breithardt G, Camm AJ, *et al*. The potential for QT prolongation and proarrhythmia by non-antiarrhythmic drugs: Clinical and regulatory implications. Report on a policy conference of the European Society of Cardiology. *Eur Heart J* 2000; **21**: 1216–1231.

18. Beuckelmann DJ, Nabauer M, Erdmann E. Alterations of K⁺ currents in isolated human ventricular myocytes from patients with terminal heart failure. *Circ Res* 1993; **73**: 379–385.

19. Waldo AL, Camm AJ, deRuyter H, *et al*. Effect of d-sotalol on mortality in patients with left ventricular dysfunction after recent and remote myocardial infarction. The SWORD Investigators. *Lancet* 1996; **348**: 7–12.

20. Torp-Pedersen C, Moller M, Bloch-Thomsen PE, *et al*. Dofetilide in patients with congestive heart failure and left ventricular dysfunction. The Danish Investigations of Arrhythmia and Mortality on Dofetilide Study Group. *N Engl J Med* 1999; **341**: 857–865.

21. Flaker GC, Blackshear JL, McBride R, *et al*. Antiarrhythmic drug therapy and cardiac mortality in atrial fibrillation. The Stroke Prevention in Atrial Fibrillation Investigators. *J Am Coll Cardiol* 1992; **20**: 527–532.

22. Grace AA, Camm AJ. Quinidine. *N Engl J Med* 1998; **338**: 35–45.

23. Pratt CM, Camm AJ, Cooper W, *et al*. Mortality in the Survival With ORal D-sotalol (SWORD) trial: Why did patients die? *Am J Cardiol* 1998; **81**: 869–876.

24. Irons D, Morrow J. The Centers for Disease Control and Prevention. Sudden death in a traveler following halofantrine administration – Togo, 2000. *JAMA* 2001; **285**: 1836.

25. Dolan M, Boyd C, Shetty G. Neuroleptic induced sudden death – a case report and critical review. *Med Sci Law* 1995; **35**: 169–174.

26. Ravin DS, Levenson JW. Fatal cardiac event following initiation of risperidone therapy. *Ann Pharmacother* 1997; **31**: 867–870.

27. Druss BG, Bradford DW, Rosenheck RA, *et al*. Mental disorders and use of cardiovascular procedures after myocardial infarction. *JAMA* 2000; **283**: 506–511.

28. Shader RI, Greenblatt DJ. Potassium, antipsychotic agents, arrhythmias, and sudden death. *J Clin Psychopharmacol* 1998; **18**: 427–428.

29. Kitayama H, Kiuchi K, Nejima J, *et al*. Long-term treatment with antipsychotic drugs in conventional doses prolonged QTc dispersion, but did not increase ventricular tachyarrhythmias in patients with schizophrenia in the absence of cardiac disease. *Eur J Clin Pharmacol* 1999; **55**: 259–262.

30. Mehtonen OP, Aranko K, Malkonen L, *et al*. A survey of sudden death associated with the use of antipsychotic or antidepressant drugs: 49 cases in Finland. *Acta Psychiatr Scand* 1991; **84**: 58–64.

31. Ray WA, Meredith S, Thapa PB, *et al*. Antipsychotics and the risk of sudden cardiac death. *Arch Gen Psychiatry* 2001; **58**: 1161–1167.

32. Zarate CA, Jr., Patel J. Sudden cardiac death and antipsychotic drugs: Do we know enough? *Arch Gen Psychiatry* 2001; **58**: 1168–1171.

33. Drolet B, Vincent F, Rail J, *et al*. Thioridazine lengthens repolarization of cardiac ventricular myocytes by blocking the delayed rectifier potassium current. *J Pharmacol Exp Ther* 1999; **288**: 1261–1268.

34. Reilly JG, Ayis SA, Ferrier IN, *et al*. QTc-interval abnormalities and psychotropic drug therapy in psychiatric patients. *Lancet* 2000; **355**: 1048–1052.

35. Buckley NA, Whyte IM, Dawson AH. Cardiotoxicity more common in thioridazine overdose than with other neuroleptics. *J Toxicol Clin Toxicol* 1995; **33**: 199–204.

36. Reilly JG, Ayis SA, Ferrier IN, *et al*. Thioridazine and sudden unexplained death in psychiatric in-patients. *Br J Psychiatry* 2002; **180**: 515–522.

37. Ray WA, Meador KG. Antipsychotics and sudden death: Is thioridazine the only bad actor? *Br J Psychiatry* 2002; **180**: 483–484.

38. Jeste DV, Gladsjo JA, Lindamer LA, *et al*. Medical comorbidity in schizophrenia. *Schizophr Bull* 1996; **22**: 413–430.

39. Druss BG, Rohrbaugh RM, Levinson CM, et al. Integrated medical care for patients with serious psychiatric illness: A randomized trial. Arch Gen Psychiatry 2001; 58: 861–868.

40. Glassman AH, Bigger JT, Jr. Prolongation of the QTc interval and antipsychotics. Am J Psychiatry 2002; 159: 1064.

41. Modai I, Hirschmann S, Rava A, et al. Sudden death in patients receiving clozapine treatment: A preliminary investigation. J Clin Psychopharmacol 2000; 20: 325–327.

42. Maisel WH, Kuntz KM, Reimold SC, et al. Risk of initiating antiarrhythmic drug therapy for atrial fibrillation in patients admitted to a university hospital. Ann Intern Med 1997; 127: 281–284.

43. Minardo JD, Heger JJ, Miles WM, et al. Clinical characteristics of patients with ventricular fibrillation during antiarrhythmic drug therapy. N Engl J Med 1988; 319: 257–262.

44. Glassman AH, O'Connor CM, Califf RM, et al. Sertraline treatment of major depression in patients with acute MI or unstable angina. JAMA 2002; 288: 701–709.

45. Carney RM, Jaffe AS. Treatment of depression following acute myocardial infarction. JAMA 2002; 288: 750–751.

46. Glassman AH, Roose SP, Bigger JT, Jr. The safety of tricyclic antidepressants in cardiac patients. Risk-benefit reconsidered. JAMA 1993; 269: 2673–2675.

47. Kane J, Honigfeld G, Singer J, et al. The Clozaril Collaborative Study Group. Clozapine for the treatment-resistant schizophrenic. A double-blind comparison with chlorpromazine. Arch Gen Psychiatry 1988; 45: 789–796.

48. Kane JM, McGlashan TH. Treatment of schizophrenia. Lancet 1995; 346: 820–825.

49. Wahlbeck K, Cheine M, Essali A, et al. Evidence of clozapine's effectiveness in schizophrenia: A systematic review and meta-analysis of randomized trials. Am J Psychiatry 1999; 156: 990–999.

50. Walker AM, Lanza LL, Arellano F, et al. Mortality in current and former users of clozapine. Epidemiology 1997; 8: 671–677.

51. Jensen VED, Gotzsche O. Allergic myocarditis seen in connection with clozapine treatment. Ugeskr Laeger 1994; 156: 4151–4152 [Abstract].

52. Lilleng P, Morild I, Hope M. Clozapine and myocarditis 1995; 115: 3026–3027 [Abstract].

53. Leo RJ, Kreeger JL, Kim KY. Cardiomyopathy associated with clozapine. Ann Pharmacother 1996; 30: 603–605.

54. Killian JG, Kerr K, Lawrence C, et al. Myocarditis and cardiomyopathy associated with clozapine. Lancet 1999; 354: 1841–1845.

55. La Grenade L, Graham D, Trontell A. Myocarditis and cardiomyopathy associated with clozapine use in the United States. N Engl J Med 2001; 345: 224–225.

56. Honigfeld G, Arellano F, Sethi J, et al. Reducing clozapine-related morbidity and mortality: 5 years of experience with the Clozaril National Registry. J Clin Psychiatry 1998; 59(Suppl 3): 3–7.

57. Warner B, Alphs L, Schaedelin J, et al. Clozapine and sudden death. Lancet 2000; 355: 842.

58. Kilian JG, Celermajer DS. Clozapine and sudden death. Lancet 2000; 355: 843.

59. Salzman MB, Valderrama E, Sood SK. Carbamazepine and fatal eosinophilic myocarditis. N Engl J Med 1997; 336: 878–879.

60. Fenoglio JJ, Jr., McAllister HA, Jr., Mullick FG. Drug related myocarditis. I. Hypersensitivity myocarditis. Hum Pathol 1981; 12: 900–907.

61. Devarajan S, Kutcher SP, Dursun SM. Clozapine and sudden death. Lancet 2000; 355: 841.

62. Roesch-Ely D, Van Einsiedel R, Kathofer S, et al. Myocarditis with quetiapine. Am J Psychiatry 2002; 159: 1607–1608.

63. Coulter DM, Bate A, Meyboom RH, et al. Antipsychotic drugs and heart muscle disorder in international pharmacovigilance: Data mining study. BMJ 2001; 322: 1207–1209.

Actions of antipsychotic drugs on ventricular action potential and ion channels

Hugh Clements-Jewery and Michael J Curtis

Cardiovascular Research, Rayne Institute, St Thomas' Hospital

London, United Kingdom

Correspondence: MJ Curtis, Cardiovascular Research, Rayne Institute,

St Thomas' Hospital, London SE1 7EH

Phone +44 (0)20 7928 9292 ext 2330

Fax +44 (0)20 7922 8139

Email Michael.curtis@kcl.ac.uk

1. Introduction

The goal of this article is to provide a molecular and cellular explanation for antipsychotic drug-induced QT widening and *torsades de pointes*. Antipsychotic drugs, like many other types of drug that evoke *torsades de pointes*, are believed to possess this 'pro-arrhythmic' action as a consequence of a mechanism unrelated to that responsible for the primary therapeutic effect (i.e., alteration of dopamine and/or serotonin neurotransmission in the central nervous system). However, this does not preclude the possibility that evocation of *torsades de pointes* is a class effect of antipsychotics, the consequence of a possible structural similarity between the ligand-recognition sites of all the relevant molecular targets (therapeutic and adverse). This article explores some of the issues that contribute to the evaluation of this possibility, especially the effects, potency, and selectivity of action on molecular targets considered relevant to *torsades de pointes*.

Drug-induced *torsades de pointes* is associated with QT widening in the ECG, the result of a specific cellular action, the widening of cardiac action potential duration (APD). If antipsychotic drugs evoke *torsades de pointes* they would be expected to do so as a consequence of APD and QT widening. If so, it is necessary that antipsychotic drugs affect specific cardiac molecular targets associated with APD widening. Most drugs that widen cardiac APD do so as a result of inhibition of a specific cardiac potassium current, I_{Kr}, which is mediated by a potassium channel encoded by the HERG gene. It is possible to widen cardiac APD by block of other potassium channels, or by delaying inactivation of sodium current (I_{Na}), but in humans the overwhelming majority of QT widening achieved by a wide range of therapeutic (and also torsadogenic) drugs is believed to be attributable to I_{Kr} block. Potassium channel block and delayed I_{Na} inactivation give rise to a corresponding increase in QT interval in the ECG. Thus, unexpected QT widening in patients taking antipsychotics is a potential cause for concern.

Drug molecular non-selectivity is, by definition, promiscuous. Unfortunately, it has not been possible to establish (for any class of drug) a simple relationship between risk of *torsades de pointes* and potency of I_{Kr} block. This is due in part to uncertainty over selectivity: the relative potency of a drug for effects on its intended molecular target versus effects on I_{Kr}, and versus actions on other molecular targets that may influence the risk of drug-induced *torsades de pointes*. With regard to the latter, it is believed that concomitant block of I_{CaL} (the current carried by cardiac L-type calcium channels) and possibly block of I_{Na}, may reduce the risk of the evocation of *torsades de pointes* by a drug that also blocks potassium channels. Thus, the full spectrum of ionic specificity and selectivity of a drug requires consideration when evaluating potential risk of *torsades de pointes*. This chapter briefly reviews the ion channels that underlie ventricular and Purkinje action potentials (AP), and discusses the consequences of blocking repolarising currents on these AP; it also summarises potencies for effects of antipsychotic drugs on cardiac potassium channels. This summary is presently incomplete due to a lack of available information.

2. Overview of drugs to be considered

Antipsychotic drugs can be delineated into 'typical', e.g. chlorpromazine and haloperidol, and 'atypical', e.g. clozapine. This article does not refer further to this delineation as it does not appear to contain any inherent pharmacological value in terms of risk of *torsades de pointes* and potency of drug action on cardiac potassium channels. Instead each drug has been evaluated individually.

3. Ventricular (and Purkinje) AP and the component currents

The ventricular AP is generated by the complex interaction between several inward and outward currents (Figure 1). By convention, any current that results in depolarisation (movement of positive charge into the cell) is defined as an inward current.

The repolarising currents that influence the shape and duration of the ventricular AP are shown in Figure 2. The terminal phase of repolarisation is associated with (and dependent on) the activity of I_{Kr}. This is why APD is particularly sensitive to blockade of I_{Kr}.

The mechanism by which drugs, including antipsychotic drugs, block I_{Kr} is shown in Figure 3. The drug must first diffuse into the cytosol via the lipid bilayer of the cell membrane, and then it must access the channel via the

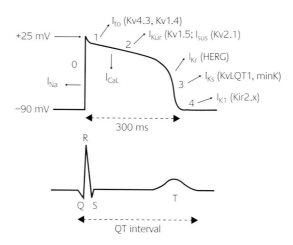

Ventricular action potential, ECG, ventricular currents and common gene names

Figure 1. The ventricular AP is labelled 0–4 to indicate its 'phases' (phase 0, rapid upstroke; phase 1, initial repolarisation; phase 2, plateau; phase 3, terminal repolarisation; phase 4, diastolic membrane potential). The currents that are active at different phases are shown. Each current is encoded by different genes (e.g. HERG for IKr) named in parentheses.

(Reproduced from Ref 1 by Brown AM, Rampe D. Drug-induced long QT syndrome: is HERG the root of all evil. *Pharmaceutical News* 7: 15–20, 2000. Taylor & Francis Ltd, http://www.tandf.co.uk/journals.)

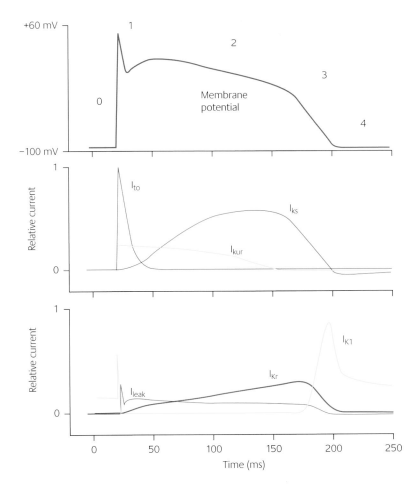

Figure 2. Potassium currents are responsible for repolarisation. An AP recorded from the mid myocardium of the ventricle is shown in representative form (top). The rapid repolarisation of phase 1 is the result of the contribution of the rapidly activating transient outward (I_{to}), the ultra-rapid delayed rectifier (I_{Kur}), and the leak (I_{leak}) currents (middle and bottom). During the plateau phase, the rapid (I_{Kr}) and slow (I_{Ks}) delayed rectifier K^+ currents, as well as I_{Kur} and I_{leak} counter the depolarizing influence of L-type calcium current (not shown). I_{Kr} and the inward rectifier K^+ current (I_{K1}) provide repolarising current during the terminal phase of the AP.

(Reprinted from Ref 24, The American Journal of Medicine, (110), Tristani-Firouzi M, Chen J, Mitcheson JS, Sanguinetti MC. Molecular biology of K^+ channel and their role in cardiac arrhythmias, pp. 50–59. Copyright 2001, with permission from Excerpta Media Inc. Original figure published in Circulation Research 1995;77(1). Zeng J, Laurita KR et al. Two components of the delayed rectifier K^+ current in ventricular myocytes of hte guinea pig type. pp 140–152. Permission granted from Lippincott, Williams and Wilkins)

Channel in resting (closed) state

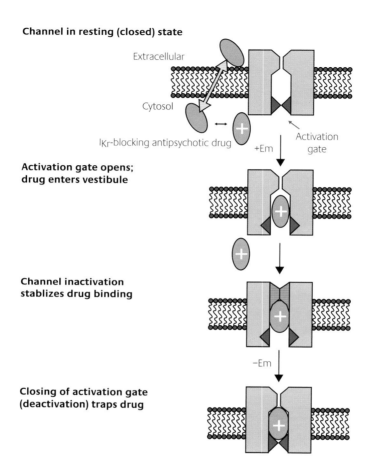

**Activation gate opens;
drug enters vestibule**

**Channel inactivation
stablizes drug binding**

**Closing of activation gate
(deactivation) traps drug**

Figure 3. Drug trapping within the K⁺ channel vestibule. I_{Kr} blocking antipsychotic drugs traverse the lipid bilayer as neutral molecules and equilibrate in the cytosol as positively charged molecules (top left). In the resting state, the activation gate (blue) of the K⁺ channel (green) remains closed. Upon depolarisation, the activation gate opens and the drug enters the vestibule to block the channel (top right). The channel then enters a long-lasting closed state (inactivation), which increases the affinity of drug binding (bottom right). Upon repolarisation, the activation gate closes (deactivation) and traps the drug within the channel vestibule (bottom left). On subsequent depolarisations, the channel is not available to conduct K⁺ ions because the drug remains bound.

(Adapted Ref 24, The American Journal of Medicine, (110), Tristani-Firouzi M, Chen J, Mitcheson JS, Sanguinetti MC. Molecular biology of K⁺ channels and their role in cardiac arrhythmias, pp. 50–59. Copyright 2001, with permission from Excerpta Medica Inc.)

cytosol. Many drugs can exist in charged and uncharged forms. This means that a drug with a pKa close to the physiological state has the most favourable properties for accessing the channel and blocking it, since appreciable lipid solubility (requiring that the drug may exist in an uncharged form) and water solubility (requiring that the drug can gain or lose charge) are each required.

4. Assessment of the meaning of drug action on the AP and currents

To demonstrate that a drug can affect a molecular target is, in itself, of little clinical value. It is a simple matter to assay and detect such a molecular action. It would be wrong, however, to deduce on the basis of this information alone that the action is responsible for the therapeutic or toxic actions of the drug on biological tissues and systems. This is because all drugs can affect more than one molecular target if the concentration of the drug is sufficiently high. Therefore, in order to make sense of the meaning and relevance of a molecular action, it is necessary to know two additional facts: the identity of all the molecular targets affected by the drug (the specificity), and the concentrations required for each effect (the selectivity). Unfortunately, with most classes of drug, especially those that have been on the market for 10 years or more, the full specificity profile, and the associated selectivity (which is always measured in terms relative to other molecular actions) are not certain. This holds true for antipsychotic drugs. Moreover, the relevance of these facts is limited by a further consideration: the range of concentrations encountered in the blood of patients to whom the drug is administered. Indeed, if a drug never reaches the concentration necessary to affect a particular molecular target, then the related cellular action is clinically irrelevant.

In order to make judgements about the implications of selectivity and specificity, numbers are required. Typically, specificity is judged on the basis of potency, which is measured as the concentration that achieves a half-maximal effect. For drugs that block receptors, this is the EC_{50} (although other related measures based upon the log-Gaussian distribution of the concentration-effect relationship may be used, such a pA2). For drugs that block channels, potency is expressed as the inhibitory concentration causing

50% block (IC_{50}). For certain types of pharmacological effects, IC_{50} is impossible to measure. In this case, arbitrary other measures are used. For APD, for example, it is theoretically possible to evoke an infinitely long AP (no repolarisation) that precludes IC_{50} determination. In such circumstances, the threshold concentration necessary for achieving a significant effect may be used instead. Selectivity, being relative, is determined by examining the EC_{50} or IC_{50} ratios between effects on different molecular targets.

5. Effects of antipsychotics on APD and cardiac potassium channels

The channels that underlie cardiac ionic currents differ in genetic origin, structure and, hence, affinity for drugs. It has been speculated that HERG shares a common structural motif with the dopamine receptors that represent the primary molecular targets for many antipsychotic drugs, although the nature of this structural motif is unknown.[1] Because of the diversity of ionic currents, and owing to the incompleteness of available data, it is not possible to establish a clear relationship between drug structure and drug action. For example, pimozide is more potent as a blocker of I_{Kr} than I_{Ks},[2] whereas sertindole is a potent blocker of both I_{Kr} and I_{Ks}.[3-4] However, it is clear from available data that all antipsychotic drugs block cardiac potassium channels, and all widen ventricular APD (see Table 1). To assess the significance of this it is necessary to consider the actions of individual drugs.

6. Consideration of individual drugs

Although this section is subdivided into sections discussing each particular drug, there are some very important cross-drug issues that arise; these issues are addressed as they emerge.

6.1 Chlorpromazine

Chlorpromazine blocks a variety of cardiac potassium channels.[5] It can be deduced that this gives rise to APD widening (although this has not been specifically investigated to our knowledge). However, chlorpromazine also blocks I_{Na}, and this effect occurs at concentrations lower than those necessary to block potassium channels.[5] This implies that any cardiovascular adverse effects of chlorpromazine are not likely to be a consequence of

Table 1. Effects of antipsychotic drugs on ventricular repolarisation and underlying potassium currents and channels.

	APD↑	HERG (I_{Kr}) (KCNH2)	Kv1.5 (I_{Kur}) (KCNA5)	KVLQT1/minK (I_{Ks}) (KCNQ1/KCNE1)	KIR2 (I_{K1})	KV4.3 (I_{to}) (KV4.3)	GIRK1/4
Chlorpromazine		s16[5]			s6.1[5]	s100[5]	
Thioridazine	^0.03[6]	^1.3[6] 0.19[15]		^14[6]			100[25]
Trifluoperazine							
Haloperidol	*0.1[4]	1[8] *0.17[4]		>>3[8]			>1000[25]
Droperidol	^0.01[9]	0.03[9]					
Flupenthixol							
Zuclopenthixol							
Pimozide	^0.1[12]	0.018[2] ^0.015[12]	>10[2]	>10[2]			>100[25]
Clozapine	*3[4]	*6[4]					300[25]
Risperidone	*0.1[4] *0.3[11]	*0.3[4] *0.03–0.3[11] **0.9[13] 0.17[15]		**>10[13]	*>30[11]	*>30[11]	
Olanzapine	1[4]	27[4] 6[15]					
Quetiapine		5.8[15]					
Sertindole	*0.3[4]	0.003–0.014[3]	2.1[3]	0.003[3]			
Sulpiride							
Amsulpride							
Ziprasidone	0.15[1]	0.17[15]					

All data are in µM and are from human channels or tissues, except *rabbit, s rat, ^guinea pig and **dog data. The gaps are the consequence of an absence of data. Values are threshold concentration for widening APD, and IC_{50} values for channel block. Note: I_{Kr} has sometimes been inferred from effects on currents after short depolarisations; and I_{Ks} inferred as current after long depolarisations. The IC_{50} values should be regarded as the more precise, since threshold effects on APD have been interpolated from most of the cited studies, and may vary in accordance with the cycle rate (which differed between studies). See references (numbered) for source material.

potassium channel block. Chlorpromazine is one of the few antipsychotic drugs to have been tested for effects on I_{K1} and I_{to}. The IC_{50} for actions on I_{K1} indicates a similar or slightly higher potency to effects on I_{Kr}, which means that if chlorpromazine blocks I_{Kr} in humans, it will do so only at concentrations that also block I_{K1}. Block of I_{K1} can lead to diastolic depolarisation, which is potentially highly arrhythmogenic. However, the IC_{50} values are among the highest of all the antipsychotic drugs studied to date, indicating that chlorpromazine is the least potent potassium channel blocker.

6.2 Thioridazine

Thioridazine has well-characterised actions on cardiac potassium channels and APD. It has ten-fold selectivity for I_{Kr} versus I_{Ks}, and its threshold concentration for widening monophasic AP in isolated guinea pig hearts is 0.03 μM.[6] The effects on APD are reverse frequency dependent[6] which is typical for drugs that widen APD as a consequence of relatively selective I_{Kr} blockade.[7] It has been suggested that I_{Kr} blockade accounts for the QT widening and torsadogenic effects of thioridazine in man, although the high plasma protein binding of this drug (99%) means that APD widening may be anticipated only when plasma concentrations are supratherapeutic, e.g. after overdosage.[6] It should be noted that its effects on APD appear to occur at a concentration 50 times lower than that required to block I_{Kr} by 50%,[4] a property shared (among a wide range of antipsychotics) only with olanzapine (this point is discussed further below).

6.3 Haloperidol

Haloperidol, like thioridazine, appears to have relative selectivity of action on I_{Kr} versus I_{Ks}.[8] However, comparison of data from separate studies reveals inconsistencies. Thus, IC_{50} for HERG block has been reported to be 1 μM in one study[8] and 0.17 μM in another.[4] In addition, data from a single laboratory found that the IC_{50} for HERG block and the threshold concentration for widening APD were largely the same.[4] These data contrast with those for thioridazine, which was found (albeit in another laboratory) to have about 100-fold selectivity for threshold APD widening versus HERG IC_{50}.[6] This disparity is intriguing. The minimum inference is that potency for HERG block may underestimate the threshold concentration for APD widening. This is an important point, as it shows that HERG block potency should not be used to predict APD widening potency (and, hence, torsadogenic potency) and that if it were shown that a drug blocked HERG at a concentration well below the therapeutic blood concentration, it would not be safe to deduce that the drug is non-torsadogenic.

There are two molecular explanations for these observations. Firstly, they may simply reflect the degree of molecular selectivity. Thus, it can be anticipated that any drug that blocks non-HERG related potassium channels at concentrations below those necessary for I_{Kr} block will inevitably widen

APD at a concentration below that which is needed for I_{Kr} block. If, for example, thioridazine was found to block I_{K1} at concentrations similar to those required for effects on APD, whereas haloperidol was found to have no effect on I_{K1}, this would provide a good explanation for the data in Table 1. Unfortunately, neither drug has been evaluated for effects on I_{K1} to date, to our knowledge. Secondly, these observations may reflect species differences, since the haloperidol data in which threshold APD and HERG IC_{50} values were similar were obtained using rabbit APD measurements,[4] whereas the thioridazine data in which the values were different (much greater potency for APD effects) were obtained using guinea-pig tissue.[6] There is no molecular basis for speculating on a species difference in I_{Kr} block, which means that between-drug variation in molecular selectivity probably offers the better explanation for these findings. This is further supported by other data from Frederiksen and colleagues,[4] discussed in the following paragraphs.

6.4 Droperidol

Droperidol has been described explicitly as a drug that widens APD as a consequence of I_{Kr} block.[9] Its concentration threshold for widening guinea-pig monophasic APD is very similar (0.01 µM) to its I_{Kr} IC_{50} (0.03 µM).[9] Given that therapeutic plasma concentrations are 0.01 − 0.4 µM,[9] some clinical APD widening may be anticipated.

The possibility of species differences in HERG/I_{Kr} block as an explanation for discrepancies between threshold APD widening concentrations and HERG/I_{Kr} block IC_{50} concentrations, is made less likely when droperidol data is contrasted with that of thioridazine. These two drugs have very similar and highly potent effects on rabbit cardiac monophasic APD, yet they differ dramatically in terms of I_{Kr} block potency (Table 1). Thus, in the same tissues from the same species (and with data from a single laboratory) droperidol was found to be only three times more potent for threshold effects on rabbit APD versus its IC_{50} for I_{Kr} blockade, whereas the potency ratio for thioridazine was 43. The best explanation for the difference between the action of thioridazine compared with droperidol is a difference in molecular selectivity (i.e. thioridazine blocks, at a very low concentration, a second potassium channel that is not blocked by droperidol). It follows from this that other discrepancies between drugs in terms of I_{Kr} block versus APD effects, are likely to result from differences in molecular selectivity rather than differences in the characteristics of the study species. This applies to the difference between haloperidol and thioridazine discussed earlier.

There are two important exceptions to any generalisation about the role of species differences in determining study outcome: (1) that APD in rat is independent of both I_{Kr} and I_{Ks},[10] and (2) that APD in rabbit is I_{Ks}-independent.[11] Thus, drugs that block I_{Ks} and I_{Kr} should not be evaluated for actions on rat APD, and drugs that block I_{Ks} should not be evaluated on rabbit APD.

6.5 Pimozide

Pimozide has consistently been reported to block I_{Kr} with an IC_{50} of $0.015 - 0.018$ µM.[2,12] In marked contrast to droperidol, haloperidol, and thioridazine, it appears to be somewhat less potent in its ability to widen monophasic APD (as determined in the guinea-pig heart) compared with its ability to block I_{Kr}.[12] However, although only a 24% prolongation of APD was reported with 0.1 µM pimozide, lower concentrations were not studied[12] so the threshold active concentration may be lower. Moreover, as with the case of other drugs that affect APD mainly by blocking I_{Kr}, pimozide's effects on APD were reverse frequency-dependent. In contrast to many other antipsychotics, there are data for pimozide's actions on several other cardiac potassium currents. Concentrations necessary for blockade of I_{Kur} and I_{Ks} were found to be beyond the clinically relevant; >10 µM.[2] Taken together these data suggest that it is likely that pimozide delays cardiac repolarisation as a consequence of relatively selective I_{Kr} blockade, as suggested previously.[12]

6.6 Clozapine

Clozapine has fairly low potency actions on APD and I_{Kr}, with threshold effects on the former and IC_{50} effects on the latter in the $3 - 6$ µM range.[4] Its action on other channels has not been studied.

6.7 Risperidone

Risperidone has consistently been found to possess threshold APD widening effects and I_{Kr} IC_{50} values in the $0.1 - 0.3$ µM range.[4,11] Of the drugs so far mentioned, risperidone is therefore qualitatively similar to clozapine and droperidol in having little within-drug variation in potency for actions on APD and I_{Kr} (although there is considerable between-drug variation in potency).

Risperidone, like chlorpromazine, has been examined for its effects on I_{K1}, I_{Ks} and I_{to}. Risperidone has little or no effect on these currents at concentrations 100 fold in excess of those affecting APD and I_{Kr}.[11,13] This means that actions on I_{K1}, I_{Ks} and I_{to} can be regarded as clinically irrelevant. Likewise, risperidone has no affect on I_{Na}.[13]

Plasma levels of risperidone can, in poor metabolisers, reach peaks of approximately 0.070 – 0.14 mM.[14] These values are approaching the IC_{50} for effects on I_{Kr} and the threshold concentration for APD widening (Table 1). The clinical relevance of this is difficult to ascertain. It is mentioned here because it illustrates a typical finding with drugs suspected of having the potential to evoke *torsades de pointes*, namely that actions necessary to explain a torsadogenic effects (actions such as I_{Kr} block) occur at a concentration not usually encountered during normal therapeutic use. The issue of whether to anticipate cardiac repolarisation problems during normal drug use, or whether to expect problems only after overdosage is therefore difficult to resolve in the absence of a large body of epidemiological data.

6.8 Olanzapine

The same investigators who evaluated clozapine have examined olanzapine. It was found to be more potent for effects on APD, but less potent for effects on I_{Kr}.[4] In this respect it shares a similarity with thioridazine. Presumably it too has potent but, as yet, unreported actions on potassium currents involved in repolarisation, such as I_{K1} and/or I_{to}.

6.9 Sertindole

Sertindole is unusually 100 times more potent in its I_{Kr} (and I_{Ks}) blocking activity compared with its APD widening activity.[3–4] This potency ratio is more extreme even than that for pimozide (Table 1) and is best explained by proposing that this drug has molecular actions on targets that lead to amelioration of APD widening. It is not clear, on the basis of presently available data what these actions may be. Unfortunately, an alternative explanation for this potency ratio is that one or more of the studies generating the data may be flawed in some respect. Further work is clearly indicated.

6.10 Other drugs and other actions

Ziprasidone appears to share with haloperidol a similar and equivalent low potency effect on HERG and APD.[1,15] Of the other drugs listed in Table 1, insufficient material is available to permit meaningful assessment of effects on APD and repolarising currents.

7. Antipsychotic-induced I_{Kr} blockade, APD widening and evocation of *torsades de pointes*

As explained earlier, if *torsades de pointes* is caused by a drug's potassium channel blocking actions, there will be concomitant APD widening. By considering the rank order of potencies for I_{Kr} blockade and APD widening, it is possible to explore whether there is a class effect of antipsychotics on APD. If so, this would allow a tentative protocol for preclinical screening for potential torsadogenic activity. Table 2 ranks available potencies for I_{Kr} blocking and APD widening effects. A relationship is apparent, although it is not 1:1. Droperidol is clearly a very potent I_{Kr} blocking and APD widening drug, whereas clozapine and olanzapine (and possible chlorpromazine) are not. However, the other drugs have actions on I_{Kr} that are not quantitatively well-related to their effects on APD. These anomalies arise because of two features: disproportionate APD widening with several drugs (thioridazine and olanzapine), and disproportionate I_{Kr} block with other drugs (pimozide and sertindole). Because data have been derived from a variety of laboratories and (in the case of the APD data) different animal species, it would be inappropriate to draw excessive conclusions. One is tempted to deduce that thioridazine and olanzapine have potent actions on potassium currents additional to I_{Kr}, whereas pimozide and sertindole may possess action on unknown cardiac molecular targets that counter their I_{Kr}-mediated effects resulting in a less than expected action on APD. This is speculative and requires further investigation. However, the data certainly argue against a predictable class relationship between I_{Kr} potency and a risk of evoking *torsades de pointes*.

Table 2. Descending rank order of potencies for antipsychotic drug-induced repolarisation delay and IKr blockade.

IC_{50} for I_{Kr} blockade	Threshold concentration for APD widening
Droperidol= Sertindole = Pimozide	Droperidol= Thioridazine
Risperidone	Sertindole = Pimozide = Risperidone = Haloperidol = Ziprasidone
Thioridazine = Haloperidol	
Clozapine= Chlorpromazine= Olanzapine	Clozapine = Olanzapine

Rank orders (most potent drugs at the top) are derived from the data in Table 1. Estimates of values that are within a margin of experimental error, (i.e. an arbitrary three fold difference in concentration) are indicated as equal in potency, in which case the drug name is followed by an equals symbol (=), indicating equal potency with the next listed drug. APD widening data for chlorpromazine and I_{Kr} blocking effects of ziprasidone are not available for assessment or inclusion in Table 1. The IC_{50} values should be regarded as the more accurate, since threshold effects on APD have been interpolated from most of the cited studies, and may vary in accordance with the cycle rate (which differed between studies). The colour coding reflects rank order of potency for I_{Kr} blockade.

A within-laboratory study has been conducted that not only relates I_{Kr} blocking potency to APD widening potency, but also quantifies an additional endpoint: evocation of early after depolarisations (EADs), that is believed by some investigators to be qualitatively predictive of a risk of evoking *torsades de pointes*.[4] These data are summarised in Table 3.

It is clear from Table 3 that it is the threshold concentration for APD widening, and not I_{Kr} potency, that best correlates with evocation of EADs. This is not unexpected, as the threshold concentration for APD widening does not correlate well with I_{Kr} blocking potency, and it is the tissue action (APD widening) rather than the molecular (e.g. I_{Kr} block) that is presumably necessary for EAD production. The same considerations may hold true for *torsades de pointes* generation. If so, this reiterates the point made earlier that I_{Kr} block is not a sine qua non for *torsades de pointes*. The large variation in APD:I_{Kr} effects ratios attests to a large variation in molecular selectivity, and it is without doubt that a tendency to evoke EADs (and perhaps also *torsades*

Table 3. Within-laboratory comparison of rank order of potencies for antipsychotic drug-induced repolarisation delay, I_{Kr} blockade and evocation of EADs.

Threshold concentration for APD widening	IC_{50} for I_{Kr} blockade	APD:I_{Kr} effects ratio	Evocation of EADs
Risperidone (0.1)	Sertindole (0.062)	Sertindole (4.8)	Risperidone 100%
Haloperidol (0.1)	Haloperidol (0.17)	Haloperidol (0.6)	Haloperidol 50%
Sertindole (0.3)	Risperidone (1.6)	Clozapine (0.5)	Olanzapine 17%
Olanzapine (1)	Clozapine (6)	Risperidone (0.06)	Clozapine 17%
Clozapine (3)	Olanzapine (27)	Olanzapine (0.037)	Sertindole 0%

Rank orders (most potent drugs at the top) are shown with µM values in parenthesis. The third column shows the ratio of the values in columns one and two. EAD data is % occurrence in groups of 6 – 7 rabbit-isolated Purkinje fibres.[4] The colour coding reflects rank order for effects on APD.

de pointes) is not one-to-one related to I_{Kr} block, and the torsadogenic effects of block of other potassium channels together with the possible ameliorating effects of concomitant actions on ICaL or I_{Na}, all factor into the ultimate expression of pro-arrhythmic effects. It is worthwhile also to note that two drugs with an even worse pharmacological profile according to this analysis were not included in the study summarized in Table 3. These are droperidol and thioridazine (see Table 2). It may be that these two drugs are the most risky of all antipsychotics in terms of torsadogenicity.

8. Pharmacokinetic considerations

A concentration of a drug may evoke experimental *torsades de pointes* or block HERG, but unless this concentration is within the range encountered in humans it has no relevance. For some drugs, including sertindole, a typical therapeutic blood concentration has not been determined. Despite this, there are data for several drugs including four of the five shown in Table 3. The important drug concentration is the steady-state free (plasma water) concentration. Seeman (2000)[16] has provided values for clozapine (0.15 µM) and haloperidol (0.0013 µM), while values for olanzapine (0.007 µM) and risperidone (7.3 µM) may be calculated from published plasma concentrations[17–18] and plasma protein binding.[19–20]

Table 4 shows that safety factor (calculated from the threshold concentration for causing APD widening, the most sensitive 'risk' factor according to Table 3) for risperidone is the closest to unity (the higher the value the lower the hypothetical safety). Moreover, there is a very good relationship between safety factor and propensity to evoke EADs. This relationship warrants further exploration with additional drugs (antipsychotic and others).

Unfortunately, the scope for overdosage in patients with schizophrenia means that typical blood concentrations may be of limited value. However, if we assume that the scope for overdosage is not drug-dependent, then the relative risks implied by the analysis here may be reasonably accurate.

9. Drug interactions

There are several classes of drug that are commonly taken therapeutically by patients also taking antipsychotics. These include antidepressants (especially lithium, tricyclics and selective serotonin reuptake inhibitors, SSRIs). These may interact either at the molecular level, or by influencing drug metabolism to enhance the effects of antipsychotics on repolarisation in the heart. For example, the metabolism of clozapine, thioridazine, haloperidol, and zupenthixol is inhibited by SSRIs[21] resulting in above-normal plasma levels. This can be expected to exacerbate the propensity of antipsychotics to evoke *torsades de pointes*. However, possible interactions with drugs commonly used in conjunction with antipsychotics are poorly characterised. At the molecular level, possible interactions between the molecular effects of antipsychotics and concomitant medication have not been adequately explored. Recently, the SSRI antidepressant, fluoxetine, was shown to inhibit human I_{Kr} with an IC_{50} of approximately 3 µM.[22] It would be interesting to

Table 4. Steady-state plasma water concentrations at therapeutic dosage in humans and its relationship to other indicators of possible adverse drug effects on repolarisation.

Steady-state plasma water concentration	Threshold concentration for APD widening	Safety factor	Evocation of EADs
Clozapine (0.15)	Risperidone (0.1)	Risperidone (0.24)	Risperidone 100%
Risperidone (0.024)	Haloperidol (0.1)	Haloperidol (0.13)	Haloperidol 50%
Haloperidol (0.0013)	Olanzapine (1)	Clozapine (0.05)	Olanzapine 17%
Olanzapine (0.007)	Clozapine (3)	Olanzapine (0.007)	Clozapine 17%

The threshold concentration for APD widening is taken from Table 3. The safety factor represents the ratio of steady-state plasma water concentration to the threshold concentration for APD widening. The EAD data is taken from Table 3.

know whether this effect occurs in a simple additive or a synergistic manner with that of antipsychotics. The effects of concomitant medication on the possible actions of antipsychotics at the level of APD widening (and possible evocation of *torsades de pointes*) are even more difficult to predict, as would be expected given the difficulty of predicting equivalent effects of individual antipsychotic drugs (see Table 3). Clearly in the clinical milieu, extensive and reliable data is inadequate, and more work is required before any sort of template for risk:benefit prediction is possible.

10. Animal models of *torsades de pointes*

A rational approach to predicting a drug's propensity to evoke *torsades de pointes* and determining the relevance of potassium channel blockade in this regard would be to relate potency for effects on ion channels to effects in animal models of *torsades de pointes*. Unfortunately, there is no clear consensus on which animal model of *torsades de pointes* is the most clinically relevant. Drugs may have torsadogenic action in one model and not another. Moreover, there is a pattern of false positives and false negatives (determined on the basis of effect with reference to perceived risk of *torsades de pointes* in man) that is not consistent between models. Thus, the present consensus is that identification of I_{Kr} blockade is of sufficient concern to make the testing of drug actions in *torsades de pointes* models redundant. This is a reasonable stance (although as noted above, failure to detect I_{Kr} block at supra-therapeutic concentrations does not preclude the possibility of *torsades de pointes* unless the drug is free from effects on other potassium currents occurring at lower concentrations). In view of this, it would be meaningless to focus here on the outcome of studies of antipsychotic drugs in animal models of *torsades de pointes*.

11. Conclusions

Where studied, antipsychotic drugs block I_{Kr} (and other potassium currents in many cases) and widen cardiac APD. They appear to do this at supra-therapeutic concentrations. However, the reports of *torsades de pointes* with antipsychotic drugs mean that I_{Kr} block cannot be ignored. To make any further judgements, particularly of an inter-drug comparative nature, would be unwise at this juncture. In an important recent article, Hondeghem and colleagues[23] examined a range of I_{Kr} blockers and found that neither I_{Kr} blockade itself nor even APD widening *per se* are the basis for pro-arrhythmia. Instead, it was the APD shape (determined by relative effects on different currents) that determines pro-arrhythmia. This study was focused primarily on evocation of ectopics, but if it can be shown to extend to *torsades de pointes*, it would tend to render much less meaningful the present obsession with I_{Kr} and APD. It is essential that actions of antipsychotics on other molecular targets including those that may protect against as well as exacerbate the probability of pro-arrhythmic actions be fully characterised.

Acknowledgements

Mi Mi Yeoh, Medical Information Specialist (Pfizer Ltd., UK) is thanked for providing literature support on antipsychotic pharmacokinetics.

References

1. Brown AM, Rampe D. Drug-Induced Long QT Syndrome: Is HERG the Root of all evil. *Pharmaceutical News* 2000; **7**: 15–20.

2. Kang J, Wang L, Cai F, *et al*. High affinity blockade of the HERG cardiac K⁺ channel by the neuroleptic pimozide. *Eur J Pharmacol* 2000; **392**: 137–40.

3. Rampe D, Murawsky MK, Grau J, *et al*. The antipsychotic agent sertindole is a high affinity antagonist of the human cardiac potassium channel HERG. *J Pharmacol Exp Ther* 1998; **286**: 788–793.

4. Frederiksen K, Adamantidis M, Matz J. Comparison of pro-arrhythmic potential of compounds with blocking effect of the HERG K⁺ channel. Proceedings Scandinavian Physiological Society meeting, University of Aarhus, II-05, 2001.

5. Kon K, Krause E, Gogelein H. Inhibition of K⁺ channels by chlorpromazine in rat ventricular myocytes. *J Pharm Exp Ther* 1994; **271**: 632–637.

6. Drolet B, Vincent F, Rail J, *et al*. Thioridazine lengthens repolarisation of cardiac ventricular myocytes by blocking the delayed rectifier potassium current. *J Pharmacol Exp Ther* 1999; **288**: 1261–1268.

7. Sanguinetti MC, Jurkiewicz NK. Two components of cardiac delayed rectifier current: Differential sensitivity to block by class III antiarrhythmic agents. *J Gen Physiol* 1990; **96**: 195–215.

8. Suessbrich H, Schonherr R, Heinemann SH, *et al*. The inhibitory effect of the antipsychotic drug haloperidol on HERG potassium channels expressed in Xenopus oocytes. *Br J Pharmacol* 1997; **120**: 968–974.

9. Drolet B, Zhang S, Deschenes D, *et al*. Droperidol lengthens cardiac repolarisation due to block of the rapid component of the delayed rectifier potassium current. *J Cardiovasc Electrophysiol* 1999; **12**: 1597–1604.

10. Rees SA, Curtis MJ. Which cardiac potassium channel subtype is the preferable target for suppression of ventricular arrhythmias? *Pharmacol Ther* 1996; **69**: 199–217.

11. Gluais P, Bastide M, Caron J, *et al*. Risperidone prolongs cardiac action potential through reduction of K⁺ currents in rabbit myocytes. *Eur J Pharmacol* 2002; **444**: 123–132.

12. Drolet B, Rousseau G, Daleau P, *et al*. Pimozide (Orap) prolongs cardiac repolarisation by blocking the rapid component of the delayed rectifier potassium current in native cardiac myocytes. *J Cardiovasc Pharmacol Ther* 2001; **6**: 255–260.

13. Magyar J, Bányász T, Bagi Z, *et al.* Electrophysiological effects of risperidone in mammalian cardiac cells. *Naunyn Schmiedeberg's Arch Pharmacol* 2002; **366**: 350–356.

14. Scordo MG, Spina E, Facciola G, *et al.* Cytochrome P450 2D6 genotype and steady state plasma levels of risperidone and 9-hydroxyrisperidone. *Psychopharmacology* 1999; **147**: 300–305.

15. Kongsamut S, Kang J, Chen X, *et al.* A comparison of the receptor binding and HERG channel affinities for a series of antipsychotic drugs. E*ur J Pharmacol* 2002; **450**: 37–41.

16. Seeman P. Dopamine Receptors: Clinical Correlates. http://www.acnp.org/g4/GN401000027/CH027.html (2000)

17. Schulz M, Schmoldt A. Therapeutic and toxic blood concentrations of more than 500 drugs. *Pharmazie* 1997; **52**: 895–911.

18. Flanagan RJ. Guidelines for the interpretation of analytical toxicology results and unit of measurement conversion factors. *Ann Clin Biochem* 1998; **35**: 261–267.

19. Eli Lilly. Summary of product characteristics – Zyprexa http://emc.vhn.net (2002)

20. Rispid product information. http://www.panacea-biotec.com/products/RISPID.htm (2002)

21. Sheline YI, Freedland KE, Carney RM. How safe are serotonin reuptake inhibitors for depression in patients with coronary heart disease? *Am J Med* 1997; **102**: 54–59.

22. Thomas D, Gut B, Wendt-Nordahl G, *et al.* The antidepressant drug fluoxetine is an inhibitor of human ether-a-go-go-related gene (HERG) potassium channels. *J Pharmacol Exp Ther* 2002; **300**: 543–548.

23. Hondeghem LM, Carlsson L, Duker G. Instability and triangulation of the action potential predict serious proarrhythmia, but action potential duration prolongation is antiarrhythmic. *Circulation* 2001; **103**: 2004–2013.

24. Tristani-Firouzi M, Chen J, Mitcheson JS, *et al.* Molecular biology of K^+ channels and their role in cardiac arrhythmias. *Am J Med* 2001; **110**: 50–59.

25. Kobayashi T, Ikeda K, Kumanishi T. Inhibition by various antipsychotic drugs of the G-protein-activated inwardly rectifying K(+) (GIRK) channels expressed in xenopus oocytes. *Br J Pharmacol* 2000; **129**: 1716–1722.

Electrocardiographic aspects of studies investigating drug-related repolarisation changes

Marek Malik

Department of Cardiological Sciences, St George's Hospital Medical School, London, United Kingdom

Correspondence: Marek Malik, Ph.D, MD, Department of Cardiological Sciences St. George's Hospital Medical School, London SW17 0RE Fax: + 44 (0)20 8725 0846 Email: m.malik@sghms.ac.uk

1. Introduction

Abnormalities of ventricular repolarisation are a serious cardiac risk factor. Clinical studies have repeatedly shown that patients with prolonged QT interval are at greater risk of cardiac mortality and malignant ventricular arrhythmias,[1-3] irrespective of whether the QT interval prolongation is caused by congenital abnormalities, or by acquired pathologies of myocardial electrophysiology. More recently, it has been also shown that similarly increased risk of cardiac arrhythmic mortality is associated with other repolarisation abnormalities such as shifts in the T wave axis,[4] increased vectorial deviation between the QRS complex and the T wave,[5] and increased localised heterogeneity of ventricular repolarisation[6] as measured by the so-called non-dipolar components.[7]

The processes of cardiac repolarisation are affected by a large number of pharmaceutical compounds. Amongst these, the most prominent are drugs that have been specifically developed for the purpose of changing cardiac repolarisation, i.e. the class III antiarrhythmic agents. Nevertheless, it has been known for decades that other non-cardiac drugs, for instance, erythromycin[8] and other anti-bacterials,[9-10] are also capable of prolonging the QT interval and modifying the electrocardiographic repolarisation patterns. Only rather recently, however, it has been fully appreciated that all drugs with active repolarisation involvement share the undesirable side-effects with antiarrhythmic drugs, i.e. they are prone to pro-rhythmic toxicity.

Understandably, observations linking *torsades de pointes* tachycardia to non-cardiac drugs[11–15] have triggered substantial interest, both from drug developers and from regulatory agencies responsible for the assessment and approval of new medicinal products.

The pre-approval assessment of potential cardiac pro-arrhythmic toxicity and the awareness of such a potential with a heterogeneous battery of different drugs is presently still a rather novel concept. Because of this, the methodology for such an assessment has not yet been fully established and different compounds frequently require specific study protocols to address the ratio between their benefit and proarrhythmic risk appropriately. Simultaneously with the advances of this field, intense discussions continue between drug developers and regulatory agencies on what is the most efficient procedure for assessing the degree of potential pro-arrhythmia. Since the field is fast evolving, it is not surprising that the regulatory agencies adopt rather strict and safe approaches and are perhaps sometimes, for good reasons, overcautious.

Considering the importance of the correct assessment of the potential of cardiac pro-arrhythmic toxicity, both for the purposes of the regulatory approval of a new drug and for its perception and acceptance among the clinical community, it is rather surprising that the electrocardiographic aspects of clinical studies investigating cardiac safety are, frequently, largely neglected. Unfortunately, as a result there are many reports in the literature of both false-positive and false-negative experiences regarding the repolarisation effects of different drugs. With this is mind, this text summarises the essential ECG requirements of clinical studies (mainly Phase I and Phase IIa) investigating cardiac pro-arrhythmic safety of new drugs. Correct appreciation of these essentials is needed, not only to plan future investigations but also to understand strengths and weaknesses of publications that report on findings in such studies.

While there are many facets to the electrocardiographic basis of QT interval and T wave related studies, this text concentrates on three key areas: (i) ECG recording; (ii) assessment of repolarisation signals and QT interval measurement; and (iii) on heart rate correction of QT interval.

2. ECG recordings

Since the incidence of *torsades de pointes* tachycardia is rather rare, even with the most repolarisation-active drugs, the outcome of clinical investigations cannot be based on the presence or absence of tachycardia episodes. Therefore, QT interval prolongation on treatment is presently accepted as a surrogate marker of potential pro-arrhythmic toxicity. It is well recognised that it is only an indirect and, therefore, rather imprecise marker. However, to date, no sufficient experience exists with other possible markers, such as the assessment of ECG morphology of repolarisation waves. Clearly, QT interval prolongation is caused by some drugs that do not have a true potential of uniquely relevant cardiac toxicity but a clear distinction between the "good", "bad" and "indifferent" QT interval prolongation is at present only theoretical. Moreover, there is no clear relationship between the extent of QT interval prolongation on treatment and degree of cardiac pro-arrhythmic toxicity. In other words, it is not true that drugs which prolong the QT interval more than others are necessarily more dangerous.[16]

For all these reasons, to evaluate this surrogate marker of pro-arrhythmic toxicity, very precise analysis of ECG signals is mandatory. To allow meaningful measurement of QT intervals and of their changes on treatment, the accuracy of ECG assessment must be substantially higher than that required in standard day-to-day clinical practice. In particular, the following points should be observed when recording ECGs in QT interval investigations, i.e. both during pre-approval studies, and during post-approval safety monitoring.

2.1 Benefits of digital ECG recordings

The ECGs should be recorded and stored digitally. While the precision (or imprecision) of standard paper printouts is fully acceptable for the most common diagnoses of ECG abnormalities (such as ischaemia, or intra-ventricular conduction abnormalities) measurement of QT interval duration in paper-printed ECGs is frequently difficult, if not directly dubious. The width of the line of ECG printout corresponds, at the standard paper speed, to approximately 10 − 15 ms, which makes the assessment of minor changes practically impossible. On the contrary, ECGs that are recorded digitally can be displayed on a computer screen in a substantial magnification, the patterns of different ECG leads can be superimposed, the voltage gain magnified, etc., all of which contribute substantially to the precision of interval measurement. Most of the contemporary electrocardiographs record the signals sampled at 500 Hz which allows a technical resolution of ± 1 ms. Moreover, the measurement of the digitally recorded signal may be stored and subsequently reviewed so that a precise record exists of the start and endpoints in the signal where the QT interval was measured.

2.2 Benefits of stationary conditions for at least 5 min

ECGs used to assess QT interval changes also have to be recorded under strict stationary conditions. This is related to heart rate correction of the QT interval, and to the so-called QT/RR hysteresis. In more detail, when heart rate accelerates or decelerates, QT interval shortens or prolongs, respectively. However, this adaptation of the QT interval duration is not instantaneous. Studies with abrupt changes in the frequency of paced rhythms have shown that approximately 2 min are needed to achieve 90% of the adaptation of QT interval following an abrupt change in heart rate.[17] Thus, if the ECG is recorded while heart rate is accelerating, the duration of QT interval is still influenced by the previously slower heart rate, thus a disparity between the QT interval duration and heart rate of the given ECG exists. In such a situation, an artificially prolonged QT interval is recorded in respect of the captured heart rate. Similarly, if heart rate is decelerating, an artificially short QT interval is recorded in respect of the heart rate of the moment.

Figure 1 shows an example of an ECG in which the duration of RR intervals is progressively changing while the duration of the QT interval is constant (the 10 sec of the recording is too short for any noticeable change in the QT interval to occur). In such an ECG, it is not at all obvious to which heart rate the measured QT interval should be related, and thus, room for substantial error exists. Consequently, ECGs showing such gradual change in heart rate must be avoided. This is best achieved when recording ECGs after the investigated subject has maintained a fully undisturbed, supine position for at least 5 min, preferably slightly longer.

3. Measurement of QT intervals

Most modern electrocardiographs report an automatic measurement of the QT interval. Such an automatic measurement is also available from many hospital-based ECG databases. Unfortunately, these automatically obtained values are usually correct only in normal noise-free recordings, where the

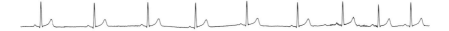

Figure 1. Example of an ECG with highly variable RR intervals but a very stable duration of QT interval. The underlying heart rate corresponding to the measured QT interval cannot be derived from this recording.

pattern of the T wave is well-defined without any morphological abnormalities. Unusual shapes of the T wave, noise in the signal, as well as confusion between T and U wave (and similarly fusions between T and P wave during faster heart rate) may easily invalidate automatic measurements. Examples of grossly inaccurate QT interval measurements are shown in Figure 2.

For this reason, no automatic algorithm can be proposed as sufficiently precise and robust to satisfy the accuracy required in the assessment of cardiac drug safety. Various combinations of manual and automatic measurements have sometimes been discussed, and advanced quality controls proposed. Still, it is much preferred to use manual measurements taken by experienced personnel. Even systems in which the ECG is firstly measured by computer and subsequently visually verified and, where necessary, corrected by human operator, do fail especially when used for massive processing of a large number of ECGs.

A particular problem of QT interval measurement is linked to the differentiation between T and U waves. The origin of U waves still remains disputed. Theories that attributed the U wave to the repolarisation of Purkinje fibres,[18] or to a combination of mechano-electrical mechanism,[19] were more recently superceded by the M-cell theory of Antzelevich and colleagues.[20] Later experiments reported by the same group, showed that pathological U waves or the so-called T/U complex is in fact a prolonged biphasic T wave with an interrupted ascending or descending limb.[21] Measurement is even less reliable for certain T/U patterns, for instance when the T wave is flat and/or inverted and the U wave augmented. A large variability of the measurement often results from complex morphology repolarisation patterns being classified differently by different observers.[22] It is very likely that electrophysiological mechanisms responsible for usual i.e.

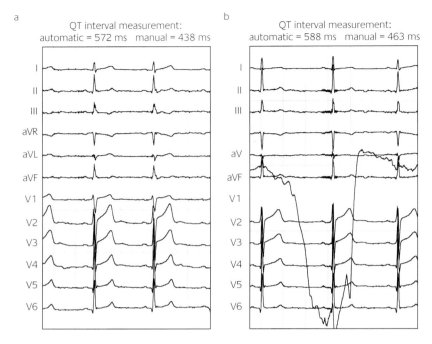

Figure 2. Two examples of errors in computer measurement of the QT interval in 12-lead ECGs. The automatic reading of both ECGs were obtained by the ECG Research Workstation by Marquette GE, which is one of the leading technical systems for ECG processing. In panel A, the computer program was probably confused by the physiologic U waves (note lead V2). The manual reading of the QT interval was 438 ms while the automatic reading showed 572 ms. In panel B, the noise in the limb leads and loss of signal in V1 probably contributed to the erroneous automatic reading of 588 ms while the manual reading was 463 ms. Each square of the display corresponds to 200 ms times 500 _V.

"physiological" U waves are different from those that lead to abnormal U waves, such as those seen in acquired long QT syndrome patients. Since all electrophysiologic signals originating from repolarisation of the ventricular myocardium constitute the T wave, the concept of biphasic or otherwise unusually shaped T wave seems to be more appropriate than the distinction between the T wave and an augmented U wave. Such a distinction may also lead to a serious underestimation of the QT interval. Indeed, augmented pathological U waves may be the only sign of adverse repolarisation changes, for instance in recordings of patients on mibefradil.[23]

A pattern resembling an augmented U wave may also originate from slow after-depolarisation. Distinction of such patterns from bizarrely shaped T waves may be very difficult, if not directly impossible. However, the signs of after-depolarisation also indicate a substantial pro-arrhythmic danger. Thus, inclusion of the after-depolarisation-related patterns resembling an augmented U wave into the QT interval is preferred. The U wave should not be incorporated within the QT interval measurement, only when there is a clear distinction between the T wave and a physiological U wave of small amplitude (mostly in frontal precordial leads). Such U waves most likely have no pathological significance and can be safely ignored.

As previously discussed, recording technology plays an important role for the precision of QT interval measurement. Some medical professionals still advocate the measurement of paper-printed ECGs using a digitising board and believe that the technical precision of the digitising equipment can be matched by human operators. Unfortunately, such assumptions are not justified, and measurement of paper-printed ECGs even when using digitising boards may lead to very substantial errors. In a study specifically designed to evaluate the human ability to operate digitising boards precisely, errors of up to 3 mm were reported in repeated measurements.[24]

Different technologies and concepts have been proposed as to which leads of the 12-lead ECG should be measured. One suggestion, mostly to reduce the cost of the measurement, is that only one lead of the 12-lead ECG should be measured. Frequently, lead II is proposed, since the longest QT interval is frequently found in that lead. Unfortunately, lead II contains the longest QT interval only in approximately 60% of normal ECGs, and in substantially fewer cases with T wave abnormalities.[16] While such a simplified approach is perhaps permissible in large Phase III studies where a somewhat compromised precision of the QT interval assessment might be acceptable, restricting the measurement to only one lead is clearly inappropriate in detailed Phase I/II studies. Following the measurement of an alternate lead, such as lead V_2 to be measured when lead II is unreadable, is also inadequate. A drug that affects the repolarisation signals may render one or other lead unreadable, allowing only inappropriate comparisons of different leads before and after treatment.

In healthy volunteers and patients without localised intra-ventricular pathologies, it is reasonable to expect that the drug effect on ventricular repolarisation will be similar in different myocardial regions (though the differential effect on endocardial, epicardial, and mid-regions should always be considered). In such a setting, measuring the QT interval in all 12 leads of the complete ECG and taking the median duration of all measurable leads seems to be the safest and most robust approach.

Since the localisation of the end of the T wave is frequently so problematic, measurement of only one single cardiac beat is not sufficient. Rather, multiple beats (e.g. 3 – 5) should be measured in each ECG, and the results of the measurements averaged. However, the selection of beats to be measured needs to be performed carefully. For instance, beats following the compensatory pause of an atrial or ventricular premature beat should be avoided because the T wave is known to be frequently abnormal in these beats. Ideally, the selection of beats for the measurement within the 10-sec ECG should not be performed manually, but should be guided by signal related criteria, e.g. by the measurement of noise pollution in the patterns of separate cardiac cycles.[25]

The question of who should measure the ECG remains controversial. The procedures proposed by the European Committee for Proprietary Medicinal Products (CPMP) specifically state that the measurement of the QT interval should be performed by electrocardiographically trained cardiologists.[26] The pharmaceutical industry frequently argues that this requirement is particularly harsh because it is both impractical and very expensive to follow. Unfortunately, there are good reasons for the CPMP requirement. When the T wave morphology is free from any abnormalities and the T wave clearly visible in a noise-free recording, the measurement of the QT interval requires only simple skills. However, pro-arrhythmic toxicity is frequently manifested by the appearance of abnormal T wave patterns including pathological U waves, unusual biphasic and semi-inverted waves. In such cases, the distinction between pathological and physiological U waves that should, and should not, be included in the measurement requires both substantial electrophysiological knowledge and clinical experience with reading the ECG lead by lead. A competence of this standard may be hard to achieve with basically trained personnel of cardiac technicians who lack the comprehensive fundamental understanding of cardiac electrophysiology.

Even when ECGs are read by qualified electrocardiologists, quality control should always be incorporated. In particular, the power calculations of every new study should include the expected precision in QT interval measurement and this precision should be verified throughout investigation. For such an assessment, two independent observers should measure a substantial proportion of the ECGs. An overall precision of interval readings quoted by clinical research organisations is frequently of very little value because it depends not only on the standard of practice of the given laboratory but also on the quality of the recorded signals and on the drug-induced changes in the morphology of T waves. These of course differ study to study, and compound to compound.

It is very regrettable that some of the clinical research organisations involved in ECG measurements for the assessment of cardiac drug safety are not very careful and/or very competent and that substantial measurement errors occur. Figure 3 shows two examples in which grossly inappropriate ECG measurement (performed by major clinical research organisations) led to serious difficulties in the evaluation of Phase I studies. Cases of such poor work are very difficult to correct. Re-measurement of potential outliers is not acceptable because every regulator will reasonably argue that errors of this kind prove the measurement to be imprecise, and that only false positive cases have been identified and corrected while possible false negative cases were ignored.

For all these reasons, it is surely preferable to follow the suggestions by the Committee for Proprietary Medicinal Products (CPMP) and to require a measurement by certified cardiologists, including an appropriate quality control. At present, there are few alternatives to such an extensive measurement approach, short of accepting the possibility of substantial errors, which may lead to grossly inappropriate decisions during the regulatory review. This may cause both a useful drug to be rejected and an unduly toxic compound approved with all the drastically undesirable consequences.

Similar precision of reading the QT interval is required when statistical analyses are based on post-approval ECG monitoring. It is unreasonable to expect that medical specialists in other fields will have the necessary experience to interpret each ECG correctly.

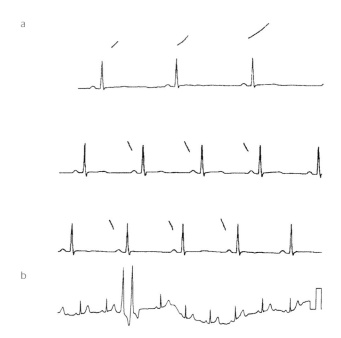

Figure 3. Two examples of poor quality of manual QT interval measurement are shown. The tracings in panel A are of lead II from serial electrocardiograms of the same subject recorded during a Phase I study. In each of these leads, the QT intervals in three cardiac complexes should have been measured. The ticks were made by an operator identifying complexes that he/she measured. Note that these include cardiac cycles in which no T-wave could have been identified. In the tracing from a different Phase I study shown in panel B, the QT interval was measured correctly but the operator included the couplet of extrasystoles into the calculation of heart rate (dividing the interval between the first and last sinus rhythm QRS complex by 9 RR intervals). This led to overestimation of heart rate and to an artificially prolonged QTc interval. In both cases, the reported QT and RR values were recorded in the study database and subsequently constituted substantial outliers with a considerable QTc interval prolongation.

4. Heart rate correction of the QT interval

A change in heart rate may occur between baseline and on-treatment ECGs not only because of the direct effect of the investigated compound on the sinus node, but also because of indirect therapeutic effects, e.g. anti-inflammatory effects when studying an anti-bacterial, autonomic conditioning due to anxiety relief, or because of a simple psychological placebo effect. Since the duration of the QT interval is profoundly dependent on heart rate, comparisons of QT intervals obtained at different heart rates are not meaningful. In some instances it has been appropriately advocated that the baseline and on-treatment heart rates should be maintained at a stable level, e.g. by atrial and/or ventricular pacing, but this approach is only suitable for very special investigations, and for ethical reasons restricted to cardiac patients who already have pacemakers implanted. In all other situations, the QT interval needs to be corrected for the underlying heart rate. In principle, such a correction is an estimation of what would have been the duration of the QT interval if the heart rate corresponded to a standard level (for historic reasons, a rather slow heart rate of 60 beats per min is used in such attempts). Thus, the principles of the correction of the QT interval are very similar to those when correcting an atmospheric pressure measured at different altitudes.

Until rather recently, simple application of one or several "universal" heart rate correction formulae (e.g. the Bazett[27] or Fridericia[28] formula) has been advocated, despite the almost universal appreciation that these formulae may substantially overcorrect or undercorrect the QT interval, particularly when heart rate is outside a narrow physiologic window.

The fact that the duration of cardiac systolic depends on heart rate was known even before the invention of electrocardiography.[29] The initial concepts of the Bazett[27] and Fridericia[28] formulae appeared in 1920. Since then, a large number of other formulae have been proposed, mainly in studies that pointed out the serious limitations of the most frequently used Bazett formula[27] and tried to replace it with a more accurate approach.[30-34] However, none of these universal formulae has been shown to operate satisfactorily in different data sets.

Each of the new proposals was based on an assumption that a "physiological" pattern of the QT/RR interval relationship exists that may be approximated by combining data of different individuals. Repeatedly, it has been overlooked in studies proposing new universal formulae that if a general physiological pattern of QT/RR relationship existed, the various studies reporting different heart rate correction approaches would not have led to such conflicting and highly variable results.

The use of a universal heart rate correction formula in any study is based on the assumption that the mathematical curve corresponding to the formula provides a reasonable fit, not only to the pooled drug-free data of the whole investigated population but also to the drug-free data of each individual participant. Such an assumption must be satisfied in order to obtain the heart rate corrected QT interval values (QTc values) that are truly independent of heart rate. QTc data need to be independent of heart rate because the comparison of on- and off-treatment recordings may otherwise be influenced by the changes in heart rate. In other words, if the QTc interval data are correlated with heart rate, both false-positive and false-negative conclusions may be reached, dependent on the change of the heart rate on treatment and on the over-correction and/or under-correction of the formula.

Although the problems of Bazett's correction with drugs that change heart rate are very well known and are frequently discussed when a drug that accelerates heart rate leads to artificial QTc prolongation, it appears that some regulators are not fully aware of the opposite possibility. For instance, it has been shown that Bazett's correction leads to a substantial and highly significant shortening of the QTc interval on beta blockers which is purely and fully related to the changes in heart rate on treatment without any noticeable heart rate-independent change in the QT interval.[35] Thus, Bazett's correction may easily mask a substantial QT interval prolongation, and important signs of pro-arrhythmic toxicity with drugs that slow heart rate. Moreover, since bradycardia is one of the pre-disposing factors of *torsades de pointes* initiation, this potential oversight may eventually have very serious consequences.

Previously proposed universal heart rate correction formulae have been derived from population data, i.e. from collections involving a large number of subjects with one or few ECG recordings in each. The possibility of recording frequent serial 12-lead ECGs in the same individual appeared only recently. Studies utilising this technology have shown convincingly that the concept of a (physiological) QT/RR relationship, that was expected to be identical in every healthy individual, is inherently flawed.[36]

Individual differences in the drug-uninfluenced QT/RR relationship are very substantial. For instance, Figure 4 shows drug uninfluenced QT/RR patterns recorded in six healthy individuals. Simple comparison of these

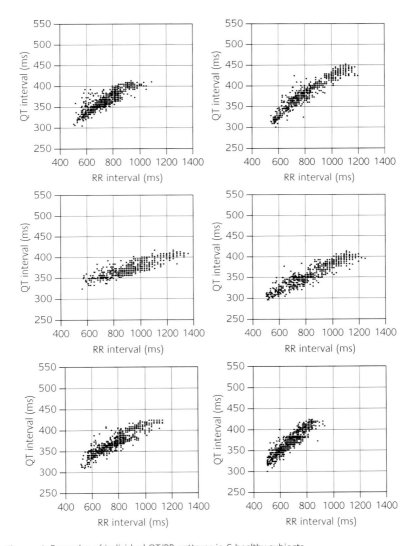

Figure 4. Examples of individual QT/RR patterns in 6 healthy subjects.

(Reproduced from Ref 36. *Heart* 2002; 87: 220–228, with permission from the BMJ Publishing Group.)

patterns shows that for instance, if the RR interval changes from 600 to
800 ms, the QT interval changes by approximately 20 ms in one subject,
while it changes by approximately 70 ms in another individual. Thus, no

mathematical formula may possibly exist that would be common to all subjects, and that would perform the heart rate correction satisfactorily in every human being.

Rather, the individual-specific drug uninfluenced QT/RR pattern needs to be established in each investigated subject in order to obtain a meaningful and unbiased method for heart rate correction. This effectively means that the mathematical form of heart rate correction will differ from subject to subject. Such an approach is methodologically valid because it has also been shown that the QT/RR relationship exhibits not only a substantial inter-subject variability but also a remarkable intra-subject stability.[37] Stability over 1 month has been reported, although unpublished data exists showing a tight reproducibility of the individual QT/RR pattern over almost 2 years (Batchvarov et al. personal communication, 2002).

In light of these observations, it seems reasonable to propose that the set-up and interplay of ionic channels that determine the duration of cardiac repolarisation and its heart rate adaptation is highly individual and probably genetically determined. For these reasons, the QT/RR relationship exhibits fingerprint-type properties in being very different between different subjects, but very stable in each individual over a prolonged time.

The need to establish a subject-specific heart rate correction formula for each study participant requires a number of drug-free ECGs to be available in each individual. Unfortunately, there is insufficient experience to derive the number of necessary recordings in each subject to construct the specific QT/RR relationship with sufficient confidence. This number depends also on the range of heart rates covered by the serial recordings. The available experience suggests that approximately 50 – 100 recordings obtained at autonomically different stages (i.e. each under standardised stationary conditions as previously described) is usually sufficient. This number is of course much larger than the number of ECGs usually obtained in standard pharmacodynamic studies. However, short of the assessment of individual QT/RR relationships, a precise heart rate correction cannot be achieved.

In some clinical situations, the individual drug-free QT/RR pattern is not obtainable for various reasons ranging from practical to ethical. For retrospective analyses of such studies, at least study-specific QT/RR patterns may be derived, practically repeating a design of a "universal" heart rate correction formula using the drug-free data in hand. While such a correction formula will ensure that no heart rate effect is projected into the QTc values of the whole population, individual outline analysis based on such a heart rate correction is not viable. (Moreover, a possibility of systematic bias exists due to the differences in the distribution of individual QT/RR patterns.)

If prospective heart rate correction of the QT interval is required, e.g. for the purposes of real-time safety assessment, both individualised and study-specific heart rate corrections are not available. In such situations, the Fridericia formula[28] seems to be a reasonable compromise. However, it must be remembered that the QTc values obtained in such a way are only very approximate, and should not be used to guide any overall conclusions.

Since it has been repeatedly shown that the Bazett formula[27] is outside the range of individual QT/RR distributions, it should never be used for purposes of drug safety assessment. Unfortunately, this invalidates substantial parts of regulatory experience, and also perhaps explains why the regulatory experience with cardiac pro-arrhythmic toxicity is so problematic.

5. Conclusions

It is very short sighted to believe that imprecise and casual approaches to ECG recordings and analysis may be tolerated in investigations of cardiac drug safety and perhaps overcome by studying larger numbers of subjects. Due to the highly individual susceptibility to drug-induced repolarisation abnormalities, the individual outlier analysis is at least as important as group mean assessment of QT interval changes. Relaxed approaches to ECG recordings and analysis can therefore both mask important positive signals, as well as lead to purely artificial concerns. Utmost precision of ECG recordings and analysis should always be required, and conclusions of studies which have not been performed in such a way should always be questioned.

References

1. Schouten EG, Dekker JM, Meppelink P, et al. QT interval prolongation predicts cardiovascular mortality in an apparently healthy population. *Circulation* 1991; **84**: 1516–1523.

2. de Bruyne MC, Hoes AW, Kors JA, et al. Prolonged QT interval predicts cardiac and all-cause mortality in the elderly. *Eur Heart J* 1999; **20**: 278–284.

3. Elming H, Holm E, Jun L, et al. The prognostic values of the QT interval and QT interval dispersion in all-cause and

cardiac mortality and morbidity in a
population of Danish citizens. *Eur Heart J*
1998; **19**: 1391–1400.

4. Kors JA, de Bruyne MC, Hoes AW, *et al*. T axis
as an indicator of risk of cardiac events in
elderly people. *Lancet* 1998; **352**: 601–604.

5. Zabel M, Acar B, Klingenheben T, *et al*.
Analysis of 12-lead T-wave morphology for
risk stratification after myocardial
infarction. *Circulation* 2000; **102**:
1252–1257.

6. Zabel M, Malik M, Hnatkova K, *et al*.
Analysis of T-wave morphology from the
12-lead electrocardiogram for prediction
of long-term prognosis in male US
veterans. *Circulation* 2002; **105**:
1066–1070.

7. Malik M, Acar B, Gang Y, *et al*. QT
dispersion does not represent
electrocardiographic interlead
heterogeneity of ventricular repolarization.
J Cardiovasc Electrophysiol 2000; **11**:
835–843.

8. Mishra A, Friedman HS, Sinha AK. The
effects of erythromycin on the
electrocardiogram. *Chest* 1999; **115**:
983–986.

9. Lipsky BA, Dorr MB, Magner DJ, *et al*.
Safety profile of sparfloxacin, a new
fluoroquinolone antibiotic. *Clin Ther* 1999;
21: 148–159.

10. Woywodt A, Grommas U, Buth W, *et al*. QT
prolongation due to roxithromycin.
Posgrad Med J 2000; **76**: 651–653.

11. Haefeli WE, Schoenenberger RA, Weiss P,
et al. Possible risk for cardiac arrhythmia
related to intravenous erythromycin.
Intensive Care Med 1992; **18**: 469–473.

12. Kemper AJ, Dunlap R, Pietro DA.
Thioridazine-induced *torsades de pointes*.
Successful therapy with isoproterenol.
JAMA 1983; **249**: 2931–2934.

13. Wilson WH, Weiler SJ. Case report of
phenothiazine-induced *torsades de
pointes*. *Am J Psychiatry* 1984; **141**:
1265–1266.

14. O'Brien JM, Rockwood RP, Suh KI.
Haloperidol-induced *torsades de pointes*.
Ann Pharmacother 1999; **33**: 1046–1050.

15. Iglesias E, Esteban E, Zabala S, *et al*.
Tiapride-induced *torsades de pointes*. *Am
J Med* 2000; **109**: 509.

16. Malik M, Camm AJ. Evaluation of drug-
induced QT interval prolongation.
Implications for drug approval and
labelling. *Drug Saf* 2001; **24**: 323–351.

17. Lau CP, Freeman AR, Fleming SJ, *et al*.
Hysteresis of the ventricular paced QT

interval in response to abrupt changes in
pacing rate. *Cardiovasc Res* 1988; **22**:
67–72.

18. Watanabe Y. Purkinje repolarization as a
possible cause of the U wave in the
electrocardiogram. *Circulation* 1975; **51**:
1030–1037.

19. Lepeschkin E. Physiologic basis of the U
wave. In Schlant RC, Hurst JW (eds).
Advances in Electrocardiography. Grune
and Stratton, New York and London, 1972,
431–447.

20. Antzelevich C, Nesterenko VV, Yan GX. The
role of M cells in acquired long QT
syndrome, U waves and *torsades de
pointes*. *J Electrocardiol* 1996; **28(Suppl)**:
131–138.

21. Yan G-Y, Antzelevich C. Cellular Basis for
the Normal T wave and the
electrocardiographic manifestations of the
long-QT syndrome. *Circulation* 1998; **98**:
1928–1936.

22. Kautzner J, Yi G, Kishore R, *et al*.
Interobserver reproducibility of QT interval
measurement and QT dispersion in
patients after acute myocardial infarction.
Ann Noninvasive Electrocardiol 1996; **1**:
363–374.

23. Benardeau A, Weissenburger J,
Hondeghem L, *et al*. Effects of the T-type
Ca(2+) channel blocker mibefradil on
repolarization of guinea pig, rabbit, dog,
monkey, and human cardiac tissue. *J
Pharmacol Exp Ther* 2000; **292**: 561–575.

24. Malik M, Bradford A. Human precision of
operating a digitizing board: Implications
for electrocardiogram measurement.
Pacing Clin Electrophysiol 1998; **21**:
1656–1662.

25. Batchvarov V, Hnatkova K, Malik M.
Assessment of noise in digital
electrocardiograms. *Pacing Clin
Electrophysiol* 2002; **25**: 499–503.

26. Committee for Proprietary Medicinal
Products (CPMP). Points to Consider: The
assessment of the potential for QT interval
prolongation by non-cardiovascular
medicinal products. The European Agency
for the Evaluation of Medicinal Products.
December, 1997.

27. Bazett JC. An analysis of time relations of
electrocardiograms. *Heart* 1920; **7**:
353–367.

28. Fridericia LS. Die Systolendauer im
Elekrokardiogramm bei normalen
Menschen und bei Herzkranken. *Acta Med
Scand* 1920; **53**: 469 – 486. [German]

29. Waller AD. A demonstration on man of

electromotive changes accompanying the heart's beat. *J Physiol* 1887; **8**: 229–235.

30. Mayeda I. On the time relation between the systolic duration of the heart and the pulse rate. *Medical Clinic of the Imperial University of Kioto* 1934; **17**: 53–55.

31. Adams W. The normal duration of the electrocardiographic ventricular complex. *J Clin Invest* 1936; **15**: 335.

32. Hodges M, Salerno D, Erlien D. Bazett's QT correction reviewed: Evidence that a linear QT correction for heart rate is better. *J Am Coll Cardiol* 1983; **1**: 694.

33. Sagie A, Larson MG, Goldberg RJ, *et al*. An improved method for adjusting the QT interval for heart rate (the Framingham study). *Am J Cardiol* 1992; **70**: 797–801.

34. Karjalainen J, Viitasalo M, Manttari M, *et al*. Relation between QT intervals and heart rates from 40 to 120 beats/min in rest electrocardiograms of men and a simple method to adjust QT interval values. *J Am Coll Cardiol* 1994; **23**: 1547–1553.

35. Malik M. The imprecision in heart rate correction may lead to artificial observations of drug induced QT interval changes. *Pacing Clin Electrophysiol* 2002; **25**: 209–216.

36. Malik M, Farbom P, Batchvarov V, *et al*. Relation between QT and RR intervals is highly individual among healthy subjects: Implications for heart rate correction of the QT interval. *Heart* 2002; **87**: 220–228.

37. Batchvarov VN, Ghuran A, Smetana P, *et al*. QT-RR relationship in healthy subjects exhibits substantial intersubject variability and high intrasubject stability. *Am J Physiol Heart Circ Physiol* 2002; **282**: H2356 – H2363.

Antipsychotic drug-induced QT interval prolongation

Simon H.L. Thomas[1] and I. Nicol Ferrier[2]

[1]Wolfson Unit of Clinical Pharmacology and [2]School of Neurology, Neurobiology and Psychiatry University of Newcastle, United Kingdom

Correspondence: Simon Thomas MD, FRCP, Wolfson Unit of Clinical Pharmacology,
University of Newcastle, Newcastle upon Tyne NE2 4HH.
Phone: +44 (0)191 222 8094 Fax: +44 (0)191 261 5733
Email: simon.thomas@ncl.ac.uk

1. Introduction

Antipsychotic drugs such as chlorpromazine and thioridazine were first introduced into clinical practice in the late 1950's and transformed the management of patients with psychosis. In the early 1960's reports emerged of a possible link between these drugs, ventricular tachycardia and sudden death.[1-3] A possible mechanism was recognised at an early stage, since ECG abnormalities indicating abnormal repolarisation were present in significant proportions of recipients.[4] These ECG effects were found to result from quinidine-like effects of the antipsychotic drug on the ventricular myocardium, specifically sodium channel blockade and delayed ventricular repolarisation.[5]

Interpretation of case reports of arrhythmia and sudden death in patients receiving these drugs is difficult because the drugs were widely used and because psychiatric patients are expected to be at a high risk of cardiovascular death in the absence of drug treatment.[6-10] This is because they have a high prevalence of risk factors for cardiovascular disease. There are also other possible mechanisms for sudden death in psychiatric patients. These include unrecognised suicide, convulsions, which may be drug induced, choking due to food bolus obstruction as a result of anticholinergic induced dry mouth, hypotension because of drug-induced cholinergic or alpha receptor antagonism, or pulmonary embolism induced by immobility in the context of prolonged retardation or stupor.

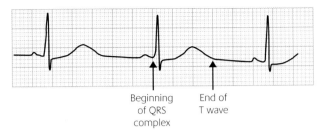

Beginning   End of
of QRS   T wave
complex

Figure 1. Antipsychotic drug-induced QT interval prolongation. The QT interval is measured from the beginning of the QRS complex to the end of the T wave (arrows). In this case the patient had taken an overdose of amisulpride. The QT interval is approximately 600 ms (3 large squares) and the heart rate 55/min (RR interval 1.090 ms). The QTc interval corrected for heart rate using Bazett's equation is 575 ms.

This chapter describes the epidemiology and risk factors for antipsychotic drug-induced prolonged ventricular repolarisation and *torsades de pointes*, drawing on experience obtained with other drugs that have similar cardiac electrophysiological effects. The risk of this adverse drug reaction is discussed and recommendations given as to how this might be minimised in psychiatric practice.

2. The QT interval and risk of arrhythmia

QT interval prolongation, reflecting prolongation of ventricular action potentials and the ventricular refractory period, may be congenital or acquired. Congenital long QT syndromes result from mutations of genes that code for specific components of cardiac ion channels. Non-drug causes of QT interval prolongation are shown in Table 1.

Prolongation of the QT interval may place the individual at increased risk of cardiac arrhythmias, particularly the characteristic polymorphic ventricular tachycardia termed '*torsades de pointes*'. However, in individuals susceptible to ventricular arrhythmias, QT prolongation may be a useful anti-arrhythmic mechanism. Drugs which prolong the QT interval, such as amiodarone and sotalol, are effective anti-arrhythmic drugs for this reason.

In healthy unmedicated subjects, the evidence linking QT prolongation with increased cardiovascular risk is conflicting. Schoeten and colleagues[11], showed an increase relative risk of all cause mortality over 15 years with QTc prolongation of 440 ms (relative risk 1.7 in men and 1.6 in women). Cardiovascular mortality

Table 1. Non-drug causes of QT interval prolongation

Bradycardia	Sinus bradycardia
	Heart block
Congenital long QT syndromes	Jervell and Lange-Nielsen syndrome
	Romano-Ward syndrome
	Sporadic
Cardiac disease	Myocardial ischaemia/infarction
	Mitral valve prolapse
	Rheumatic fever
	Myocarditis
	Bundle branch block
Metabolic abnormalities	Hypocalcaemia
	Hypothyroidism
	Hypokalaemia
	Hypomagnesaemia
Intracranial pathology	Head injury
	Subarachnoid haemorrhage
Others	Low energy diets
	Anorexia nervosa
	Alcoholism

largely accounted for this increase in risk. Conversely, Goldberg and colleagues[12] showed no statistically significant increase in overall relative risk of death (relative risk 1.02, 95% Confidence Interval [CI] 0.70 – 1.49), or sudden death (relative risk 1.31, 95% CI 0.60 – 2.86) in patients with QTc interval > 0.44 sec in data derived from the Framingham Heart Study. However, a clinically relevant increase in risk of sudden death cannot be excluded based on these data. There is no epidemiological evidence dealing with the risks associated with more pronounced QT prolongation. In a study involving almost 2,000 patients with congenital long QT syndrome and their relatives, 52% of affected probands, 22% of affected relatives, and 0% of unaffected relatives had a QTc interval of more than 500 ms. The risk of a cardiac event increased by an average of 5.2% (95% CI 1.7, 8.8%) for every 10 ms increase in QTc.[13]

In patients with cardiovascular disease there is better evidence that QT prolongation is associated with increased risk of arrhythmia or death, such as in acute myocardial infarction (although not all published research supports a link), and in patients referred for 24 hour Holter monitoring. A link has also been demonstrated for patients with liver disease. These issues are reviewed in more detail elsewhere.[14] It is not clear if all the increased risk is attributable to the prolongation of the QT interval and hence ventricular repolarisation, or whether the latter is partly a reflection of the extent of heart disease suffered by the individual.

3. Drug induced QT prolongation

An ever increasing number of drugs have been associated with QT prolongation and the majority of these have also caused *torsades de pointes* ventricular tachycardia (Table 2). The mechanism of QT prolongation has been investigated for many of these drugs. The most important of these is via blockade of the delayed rectifier potassium channel I_{Kr}; this blockade prevents the outward movement of potassium that is responsible for ventricular depolarisation. With the exception of anti-arrhythmic drugs, this is an entirely separate mechanism from their primary pharmacological action. This is an important point: since potassium channel blockade is not required for these drugs to exhibit their beneficial effects, a risk of arrhythmia is entailed which is not associated with any clinical advantage.

4. Factors affecting the risk of drug induced arrhythmia
4.1 The clinical characteristics of the subject

Patients who have abnormal ventricular repolarisation in advance of drug therapy are probably at increased risk of developing arrhythmia when started on drugs that further prolong repolarisation. Indicators of abnormal repolarisation include abnormalities of the T wave or large U waves, as well as QT prolongation. Patients who have had previous episodes of *torsades de pointes*, drug-induced or not, are at particular risk. Patients with pre-existing cardiac disease such as left ventricular dysfunction or hypertrophy, are also at increased risk, as are recipients of digoxin. *Torsades de pointes* is most likely to occur when the heart rate is slow and in the presence of extrasystoles. Conditions associated with these factors, such as heart block, increase the risk of *torsades de pointes*. This can be reduced by increasing the underlying heart rate. The arrhythmia is more likely to occur in the presence of electrolyte abnormalities, such as hypokalaemia, hypocalcaemia or hypomagnasemia. Treatment with diuretics appears to increase risk, perhaps by producing such electrolyte abnormalities.[15–16]

Table 2. Some drugs causing QT prolongation

Anti-dysrhythmic drugs		
Class Ia	Quinidine	Procainamide
	Disopyramide	Propafenone
Class III	Amiodarone	Sotalol
	d-sotalol[1]	Ibutilide[1]
	Almokalant[1]	Dofetilide
Calcium channel blockers	Prenylamine[2]	Terodiline[2]
	Mibefeadil[4]	
Psychiatric drugs	Thioridazine[3]	Pimozide[3]
	Sertindole[3]	Ziprazidone[1]
	Chlorpromazine	Haloperidol
	Tricyclic antidepressants	Citalopram
	Lithium	Chloral hydrate
	Levacetylmethadol[1]	
Antihistamines	Terfenadine[3]	Astemizole[3]
Antimicrobial and antimalarial drugs	Erythromycin	Clarithromycin
	Spiramycin	Clindamycin
	Trimethoprim-sulphamethoxazole	Pentamidine
		Quinine
	Chloroquine	Halofantrine
	Amantadine	Moxifloxacin[3]
	Sparfloxacin[3]	Grepafloxacin[2]
	Ketoconazole	
Serotonin antagonists	Ketanserin[1]	Cisapride[2]
Others	Organophosphates	Probucol[2]
	Tacrolimus	Indapamide
	Amrinone[1]	Milrinone[1]
	Arsenic	Vasopressin
	Fosphenytoin	

[1]not marketed in the UK
[2]withdrawn due to pro-arrhythmia
[3]alterations in licensing as a result of QT prolongation/pro-arrhythmia
[4]withdrawn for other reasons

Patients with chronic alcoholism may be at increased risk because this may be associated with liver disease which increases the risk of sudden death.[17] The impact of other recreational substances on cardiac repolarisation and sudden cardiac death is unclear. QT interval prolongation has been reported with ecstasy[18] and cocaine,[19] and sympathomimetic agents may increase the risk of ventricular arrhythmias independent of any effects on repolarisation. However, there are little published data in this area and further research is needed.

Women have a longer QT interval on average than men[20-21] and epidemiological studies have consistently shown that a disproportionate number of episodes of drug induced *torsades de pointes* occur in women.[22] The reason for this difference in risk has not been fully elucidated but there is evidence that sex steroids effect the numbers and function of potassium channels in cardiac membranes.[23]

A group combining several risk factors are patients with anorexia nervosa. These are at increased risk, not only because they are usually female and often have electrolyte abnormalities, but also because, relative to their low body weight, high doses of antipsychotic drugs are often employed.

4.2 The extent of QT prolongation

The relationship between the degree of drug-induced QT interval prolongation and the extent of the increase in risk of arrhythmia has not been subject to formal epidemiological study. However, risk appears to increase with more extreme QT interval prolongation. *Torsades de pointes* appears unusual if the QT interval is less than 500 ms, and in one study the mean QT interval prior to the onset of *torsades de pointes* was 580 ms.[24] The relationship between the extent of drug-induced QT prolongation and risk of *torsades de pointes* is discussed in more detail in other chapters.

4.3 Properties of the drug

Some drugs are more potent than others at producing QT interval prolongation and arrhythmias at therapeutic doses. This depends on their relative potency for producing their clinically intended effect compared with their potency at provoking QT interval prolongation. Blockade of cardiac ion channels is a stereoselective process and for drugs with a chiral centre QT prolongation may be dependent on the enantiomer being used. For example, the QT prolongation caused by racemic terodiline appears to be exclusively associated with the R(+) enantiomer,[25] and there is also evidence for stereoselective effects on potassium channels or *torsades de pointes* for R(+)-halofantrine, R(+)-bupivacaine and R(+)-levoacetylmethadol.[26]

It is likely that drugs which produce the same degree of QT prolongation may provide different risks of arrhythmia. For example, it is generally believed that the class III antiarrhythmic drug amiodarone, is less commonly associated with *torsades de pointes* than other drugs, even though it causes QT prolongation which is just as marked.[27–28]

Why some drugs that cause QT prolongation may be safer than others is an important question for further research. The electrophysiological properties of the drug are important; for example, its propensity to prolong the action potential and to produce triggered activity, including early after-depolarisations and *torsades de pointes* in animal models. In the presence of some drugs it may be very difficult to produce triggered activity and *torsades de pointes*, despite marked action potential prolongation. An example is sertindole.[29] It remains to be established how predictive such studies are of arrhythmias during the clinical use of the drug. Those drugs which produce heterogeneous prolongation of QT interval across the myocardium (increased QT dispersion) may carry a higher risk, compared with those which produce a homogeneous QT prolongation.[28]

Some drugs have ancillary properties that may either increase of decrease the risk of arrhythmia. For example, drugs that are associated with tachycardia may be less likely to produce *torsades de pointes*, since this occurs most often when the heart rate is slow.[30]

There is also evidence that *torsades de pointes* most often occurs disproportionately early during therapy, at least with quinidine.[16,31–32] If this observation is true for other drugs it has implications for monitoring, since it would be logical to focus this at the time of highest risk.

4.4 Drug concentration

There is ample evidence that QT prolongation and resulting arrhythmias are concentration-related effects. Recent epidemiological studies in psychiatric patients have confirmed this association.[33–35] Any factor that increases drug concentration at the site of action will increase risk. Examples are discussed below.

4.4.1 Drug overdose

Arrhythmia is more common in patients who are also taking other drugs that cause QT prolongation or who are given high therapeutic doses of these drugs.[36] The latter should be avoided unless there is sufficient clinical justification.

4.4.2 Impaired drug clearance

Impaired hepatic and renal function may enhance plasma and tissue drug concentrations and substantial QT interval prolongation may occur with resulting risk of arrhythmia. For example, QT prolongation is more marked in recipients of sotalol who also have impaired renal function.[37]

There are genetic polymorphisms for some hepatic p450 oxidative enzymes and for N-acetyl transferase (Table 3). Some of these enzymes are responsible for the metabolism of drugs that cause QT prolongation and *torsades de pointes*. As a result, some patients who do not express individual isoforms may experience enhanced (parent drug causes QT prolongation) or attenuated (metabolite causes QT prolongation) ECG effects. For example, the class Ia antiarrhythmic drug procainamide is acetylated to the active metabolite n-acetyl procainamide (NAPA), which is more potent than the parent drug at prolonging repolarisation. This metabolism is delayed in slow acetylators who may therefore be less likely to develop QT interval prolongation.[38] Similarly, the class Ic agent encainide is converted to its metabolite 3-methyl O-desmethyl encainide (MODE) by the hepatic p450 isoform CYP2D6 (debrisoquine hydroxylase). MODE causes QT prolongation which is thus observed in rapid but not slow hydroxylators.[39] There is, as yet, no direct clinical evidence that failure to express hepatic enzymes predisposes the individual to arrhythmia. However, this is an important area for further research since it offers the possibility of identifying patients at increased risk before drug exposure.

Pharmacogenetic factors are relevant to antipsychotic drug therapy as several antipsychotic and antidepressant drugs are hydroxylated via CYP2D6 (debrisoquine hydroxylase). Thioridazine is an important example. Slow hydroxylators of debrisoquine achieve higher plasma concentrations of the parent drug and its ring sulphoxide metabolite than rapid hydroxylators,[40] and thioridazine-induced QT prolongation has been linked to plasma concentration.[41] A summary of the metabolising enzymes, genetic polymorphisms and enzyme inhibitors relevant to QT-prolonging psychoactive drugs is given in Table 3.

Table 3. Important enzymes in the metabolism of psychotropic and other QT prolonging drugs. Psychotropic drugs are shown in italics and drugs that commonly cause QT interval prolongation are marked with an asterisk.[60-64]

Enzyme	Poly-morphism	Probe drugs	Poor metaboliser phenotype frequency	Important substrates	Important inhibitors
CYP1A2	Yes	Caffeine	12%	*Clozapine*	*Fluvoxamine*
				*Haloperidol**	Ciprofloxacin
				Amitriptyline	
				Clomipramine	
				*Imipramine**	
				Maprotiline	
				Fluvoxamine	
				Propranolol	
				Theophylline	
				Methadone	
CYP2D6	Yes	Debrisoquine	5–10%	*Thioridazine**	Paroxetine
		Sparteine	(Caucasians)	*Haloperidol**	Fluoxetine
		Dextromethor-phan	0.2–1%	*Chlorpromazine**	Norfluoxetine
			(Asians and blacks)	*Perphenazine*	*Thioridazine**
				Zuclopenthixol	Sertraline
				Risperidone	Halofantrine*
				*Sertindole**	Chloroquine*
				Clozapine	Quinidine*
				*Amitriptyline**	Propafenone*
				*Clomipramine**	
				*Desipramine**	
				*Imipramine**	
				*Nortriptyline**	
				Fluoxetine	
				Fluvoxamine	
				Mianserin	
				Venlafaxine	
				Maprotiline	
				Bupropion	
				Encainide	
				Flecainide	
				Propafenone	
				Mexilitine	
				Metoprolol	
				Codeine	
				Tramadol	
CYP2C9	Yes	Tolbutamide	1–3%	Diclofenac	*Fluoxetine*
				Ibuprofen	
				Naproxen	
				Phenytoin	
				Warfarin	
				Tolbutamide	

Table 3. continued

Enzyme	Poly-morphism	Probe drugs	Poor metaboliser phenotype frequency	Important substrates	Important inhibitors
CYP2C19	Yes	S-mephenytoin Omeprazole	3–6% (Caucasians and blacks) 15–30% (Asians)	*Hexobarbital* *Diazepam* *Citalopram** *Imipramine** *Clomipramine** *Amitriptyline** *Moclobemide* Omeprazole Propranolol	*Fluvoxamine* *Fluoxetine* *Sertraline (?)* *Clozapine (?)* Omeprazole
CYP3A4	No	Nifedipine	–	*Carbamazepine* *Alprazolam* *Triazolam* *Zolpidem* *Risperidone* *Quetiapine* *Pimozide** *Sertraline* *Venlafaxine* *Fluoxetine* *Desipramine** *Imipramine** *Nortriptyline** *Terfenadine** Propafenone* Quinidine* Diltiazem Midazolam	*Fluvoxamine* *Nefazodone* *Fluoxetine* *Sertraline* Erythromycin Clarithromycin Troleandomycin Ketoconazole Itraconazole Cimetidine Indinavir Ritonavir, Saquinavir Grapefruit juice
N-acetyl transferase	Yes		60% (Caucasians) 15% (Asians) 5% (Inuit)	*Phenelzine* Procainamide* Hydralazine Sulphonamides Isoniazid	

There is an increased risk of provoking arrhythmia in some subjects if the metabolism of the drug is highly variable between individuals. Individuals with comparatively slow metabolism or excretion are at risk of unusually high plasma and tissue drug concentrations and marked QT prolongation in spite of the use of modest drug doses. If the elimination half-life is long there is a risk of accumulation in susceptible groups, particularly the elderly. Terodiline, a drug used to treat urinary incontinence, had these pharmacokinetic characteristics and was associated with a large number of arrhythmias and episodes of cardiac arrest in elderly recipients before it was withdrawn.[42–43]

4.5 Drug interactions

Pharmacokinetic drug interactions resulting in increased plasma or tissue concentrations of a QT interval prolonging drug are a particularly important source of *torsades de pointes*. The most common interaction is via inhibition of the hepatic cytochrome p450 isoform CYP3A4. This isoform is important because it is very abundant in human liver and is primarily responsible for the metabolism of many QT prolonging drugs. Other cytochrome p450 isoforms are also subject to inhibition; important inhibitors for these enzymes are shown in Table 3.

The most important pharmacodynamic interaction is from the combined use of two drugs that prolong ventricular repolarisation, since these may have an additive affect on QT interval. It is important to note that some hepatic enzyme inhibitors (e.g. erythromycin, ketoconazole) also delay cardiac repolarisation and this effect increases the severity of the interaction. Drugs that cause electrolyte abnormalities, such as hypokalaemia, also increase risk. Diuretics are the most common example.

In the context of antipsychotic drug therapy, there is increasing evidence of significant interaction with selective serotonin reuptake inhibitors and tricyclic antidepressants. Interaction with the latter is probably of particular importance since these drugs also produce QT prolongation independently. There is also emerging evidence of a link between dosulepin (dothiepin) use and ischaemic heart disease[44] which, if confirmed, would further augment the risk of sudden death.

Experience with terfenadine, the non-sedating antihistamine, illustrates the importance of some of these issues. The drug provides its H_1 antihistamine actions via an active metabolite, terfenadine carboxylate (fexofenadine), which does not affect the QT interval. The parent drug causes prolongation of the QT interval, but in most subjects this is minor because of rapid hepatic conversion of terfenadine to fexofenadine by the hepatic p450 isoform CYP3A4. However, in the presence of drugs or other substances which inhibit CYP3A4, the QT interval may become prolonged to a dangerous extent and *torsades de pointes* may be precipitated. *Torsades de pointes* may also occur because of liver disease or terfenadine overdose, including the use of high therapeutic doses.[45–46]

Another non-sedating antihistamine, astemizole, and the prokinetic drug, cisapride, have also been withdrawn due to their association with QT prolongation and ventricular arrhythmias. As with terfenadine, interactions with CYP3A4 inhibitors have been implicated for both drugs.[47] A similar interaction precipitating *torsades de pointes* has been described between pimozide and clarithromycin.[48]

4.6 The circumstances of drug administration

Several of the case reports of sudden death involve agitated patients undergoing restraint.[49–50] Concerns have been raised that patients may be at increased risk of arrhythmia during such physiological activation, as a result of increased sympathomimetic activity. To date, epidemiological studies suggest that, if this mechanism exists, it is uncommon.[51]

5. Differential toxicity of antipsychotic drugs

Evidence has been available for some time suggesting that the pro-arrhythmic actions of antipsychotic drugs vary, with some agents being particularly potent at causing arrhythmias and sudden death.

A disproportionate number of case reports of arrhythmia or sudden death have involved thioridazine, and doses of 100 mg daily or more caused QT interval abnormalities in over half of the recipients. A study in Finland of 49 cases of sudden death affecting patients taking psychiatric drugs found that 46 were exposed to a phenothiazine and in 28 cases, specifically, thioridazine. The study concluded that this finding was out of proportion compared with the local use of the drug.[52]

Reports of 13 sudden deaths in recipients of pimozide prompted the UK Committee on Safety of Medicines (CSM) to issue specific recommendations on the use of this drug, including gradual dose escalation, recording an ECG before and periodically during treatment in those receiving high doses. Affected patients were often receiving high doses of pimozide or concurrent treatment with other neuroleptic drugs. In view of the long and variable plasma half-life of the drug, rapid dose escalation may have caused drug accumulation and toxicity.

More recently the atypical antipsychotic drug sertindole was linked with QT interval prolongation, with 36 suspected fatal adverse drug reactions and 13 episodes of serious but non-fatal arrhythmias reported.[53] The drug was withdrawn by the manufacturers in 1998. However, restrictions in the European Union were lifted in June 2002 following the receipt of reassuring epidemiological and *in vitro* data.

Although this evidence suggested that the risk of arrhythmia may differ between antipsychotic drugs, it has only been confirmed recently by systematically collected epidemiological data, discussed further below.

5.1 Effects on the ECG

Early studies of the ECG effects of antipsychotic drugs were limited by their small size, making it difficult to draw reliable conclusions about differential effects of drugs and dose response. Three recent studies have provided substantial additional information.

Warner and colleagues, performed ECGs in 111 patients receiving neuroleptic therapy, as well as 42 untreated controls.[33] QTc prolongation (defined as > 420 ms) was more common in the treated patients, and particularly in those taking high doses (more than 2000 mg chlorpromazine equivalents), although the study was too small to provide information on the differential effects of individual drugs.

To investigate the possible differential cardiotoxic effects of antipsychotic drugs, ECGs were collected from 495 psychiatric patients in various in-patient and community settings in the north-east of England.[34] Details of their clinical histories and drug treatment were taken, together with a 12-lead ECG. Normal limits for ECG variables were defined from a reference group of 101 healthy individuals. Logistic regression was used to investigate factors predictive of QTc prolongation. These factors were found to be: age over 65 years, use of tricyclic antidepressants, and use of either thioridazine or droperidol. For antipsychotic drugs as a whole, the risk of QT prolongation was significantly greater if high or very high doses were used, compared with low doses. This relationship persisted even if thioridazine and droperidol recipients were excluded from the analysis. For thioridazine, QT prolongation was more common in recipients of more than 600 mg daily. Significant relationships between QT interval prolongation and other individual antipsychotic drugs were not found, although could not be excluded for many drugs because of their low level of exposure in this population. Because of the time period over which the study was conducted, the numbers of patients taking newer atypical antipsychotic drugs was too small for conclusions about these to be drawn.

These data suggesting differential effects of antipsychotic drugs on the QT interval are supported by the Pfizer 054 study, a randomised open parallel comparison of the effects of six antipsychotic drugs on the QT interval at steady state in 185 patients with stable psychotic disorders. Drugs were introduced after tapering of previous medication and a five-day placebo run-in. The largest mean increases in QTc interval were seen with thioridazine 150 mg twice daily (35.6 ms), while changes with ziprasidone 80 mg twice daily (20.3 ms), quetiapine (14.5 ms), risperidone (11.6 ms) olanzapine (6.8 ms), and haloperidol 15 mg daily (4.7 ms) were less marked.[54]

5.2 Effects on sudden deaths

Ray and colleagues, have recently investigated the rates of sudden cardiac death in Tennessee Medicaid enrollees aged 15 – 84 years without life-threatening non-cardiac illness between 1988 and 1993.[35] The cohort comprised 481,744 persons, 1.3 million person years of follow-up (including 53,614 of current antipsychotic drug use) and a total of 1,487 sudden cardiac deaths. In the unexposed group there were 11.3 deaths per 10^4 person years of follow-up. This figure increased to 14.4 and 26.9 per 10^4 person years for current users of low and high doses, respectively, defined as less than or greater than 100 mg thioridazine equivalents. Multivariate-adjusted risk of death was increased 2.4 times in recipients of antipsychotic drugs. Risk was highest with thiothixene (RR 4.23, 95% CI 2.00 – 8.91), chlorpromazine (3.64, 95% CI 1.36 – 9.74), thioridazine (3.19, 95% CI 1.32 – 7.68), and haloperidol (1.90, 95% CI 1.10 – 3.30).

A case-control epidemiological study was performed in the north-east of England to investigate the link between sudden death and drug therapy.[51] A retrospective notes review was conducted of all in-patient deaths occurring in five psychiatric hospitals over the 12 years between 1984 and 1995. Sudden deaths were defined as deaths occurring within one hour of the patient being observed in their usual state of health, or found dead more than one hour after having been seen but having been seen in their usual state of health within the last 24 hours. Patients with a proven non-cardiac cause or acute myocardial infarction were excluded. Of 1,202 deaths reviewed, 77 (6.4%) met these criteria for sudden death. Most of these patients were elderly (median age 69 years) and most had been in hospital for more than one year (median duration of admission 633 days). To investigate for a possible contribution from drug therapy, these patients were matched to controls on the basis of sex, age (five-year age bands) and duration of admission. One control was also matched for primary psychiatric diagnosis.

Using conditional logistic regression, factors associated with sudden death included: the presence of an organic psychiatric disorder, the presence of hypertension or previous myocardial infarction, and treatment with thioridazine. The association with thioridazine was robust and persisted whether one or other or both controls were used in the statistical analysis. No relationship between sudden death and thioridazine dose was observed in this comparatively small study. There were inadequate data to draw conclusions for a possible link between droperidol and sudden death.

Although this study is comparatively small and retrospective, its result raised serious concerns about the safety of thioridazine, particularly when viewed in the presence of the other epidemiological evidence. Thioridazine is a potent blocker of the delayed rectifier potassium channel[55] and has been shown to be more toxic than other antipsychotic drugs when taken in overdose.[56] These data have resulted in regulatory changes which have severely restricted indications for thioridazine in both the UK and USA. The manufacturers of droperidol have suspended marketing of this product.

The epidemiological studies described above were all conducted before the widespread introduction of atypical antipsychotic drugs, with the exception of clozapine, and provide no evidence about their relative safety. A further case-control study is currently underway in the UK which may provide information on more recently introduced drugs.[57]

6. Putting the risk in perspective

In order to estimate the risk of sudden death attributable to a drug using an odds ratio obtained from a case-control study, an estimate of the absolute risk of sudden death in an unmedicated population is needed. Three recent epidemiological studies have estimated the underlying crude risk of sudden death per 10,000 patient years in individuals without apparent cardiovascular disease as 5.5 (males aged 40 – 84 years at baseline and follow-up for 12 years)[58], 7.2 (aged 43 – 52 years, follow-up 23 years)[59] and 11.3 (Medicaid enrollees aged 15 – 84 years).[35]

The Medicaid data provide an estimate of the overall additional risk of sudden death attributable to high doses of antipsychotic drugs as 15.6 deaths per 10^4 patient years of treatment.[35] A higher risk would be expected for more toxic drugs. For example, if thioridazine increases the risk of sudden death approximately six-fold, as suggested by the Newcastle data, the absolute increase in risk of sudden death with this drug would be between 25 and 40 per 10,000 patient years, depending on the underlying rate of sudden death being used.[51] Thus, although this drug appears the most potent of the traditional antipsychotic drugs in causing this effect, the absolute risk to recipients in real terms is comparatively small in an otherwise healthy population. However, attributable risks would be substantially higher in patients with increased underlying level of risk due to age or heart disease or other risk factors. These include: increased body mass index, smoking, diabetes, parental history of sudden death, and increases in heart rate, blood pressure or cholesterol.[59] Such patients were often prescribed the drug until recent changes were made regarding the licensing of thioridazine.

7. Minimising risk of sudden death with antipsychotic drugs

Although the risk of sudden death with antipsychotic drugs is small, it is important that all reasonable steps are taken to minimise the risk of this devastating adverse drug reaction. In the first instance, it is important that attention should be paid to the general health of patients with psychosis, since reduction in the prevalence of heart disease will reduce the intrinsic risk of sudden death, as well as the risk of drug-induced arrhythmia. Modifiable risk factors for ischaemic heart disease should be identified and managed appropriately, including smoking, hypertension, hyperlipidaemia, sedentary lifestyle and obesity. It is important to recognise that obesity, hyperlipidaemia and glucose intolerance may be exacerbated by antipsychotic drug therapy,[60] and in some cases this may be a more important risk for the patient than that of *torsades de pointes*.

The choice of antipsychotic therapy is important in determining risk. The use of drugs with more pronounced effects on cardiac repolarisation can only be justified if the drug has specific advantages for the patient in comparison with antipsychotic drugs with less marked electrophysiological risks. High doses and drug combinations should only be used when there is a clinical justification, particularly if the combination may result in inhibition of clearance or additive ECG effects.

To further reduce the risk of arrhythmia, all patients should be assessed for cardiovascular disease prior to the institution of antipsychotic drug therapy. This should, whenever possible, include an ECG, which should be examined for evidence of ischaemic heart disease, left ventricular hypertrophy and repolarisation abnormalities. The presence of such factors may affect the choice of antipsychotic drug chosen or increase the frequency of monitoring required, as well as prompt a more detailed cardiac assessment. An ECG prior to antipsychotic therapy is particularly important if higher risk antipsychotic drug treatment is contemplated (e.g. thioridazine, sertindole, and pimozide), if high dose or parenteral antipsychotic drug therapy is to be used, or in people with a history of cardiovascular disease. It is also prudent to check the blood biochemistry, particularly plasma potassium, before embarking on such therapy, especially in patients at higher risk of electrolyte abnormalities due, for example, to anorexia nervosa, diuretic use, or dehydration.

Periodic monitoring of the ECG and electrolytes during therapy is increasingly being advocated when high risk antipsychotic drug therapy is to be used. The most recent Maudsley guidelines[61] recommend continuous ECG monitoring following the administration of parenteral antipsychotic therapy, especially when higher doses are used. The summaries of product characteristics of several higher risk drugs recommend periodic ECG monitoring during therapy, which should also be considered in patients at increased risk because of underlying heart disease. However, if ECGs are to be done, it is not clear how often this should occur and whether this would have any impact on cardiac mortality. A case can be made for these to be performed every few days following initiation of therapy or dose escalation until steady state concentrations are thought to have been reached, bearing in mind the experience with quinidine, when the median time between institution of therapy and *torsades de pointes* was only three days.[32] Thereafter ECG and electrolyte assessment could be recommended every few months, at times of acute illness, when potentially interacting drugs are introduced, or if the patient experiences symptoms that could be due to arrhythmia, e.g. syncope or fits. Although such monitoring may help prevent some episodes of drug-induced *torsades de pointes*, the numbers prevented will be very small in comparison with the huge numbers of ECG and blood tests required, and the cost-effectiveness of this approach is very uncertain. Further research is needed before such an approach is widely adopted.

A major source of drug-induced arrhythmia is from drug interactions, and strategies are needed to minimise the risk of these interactions. One suggestion has been that the patient should carry a warning card listing the risk factors, precautions and contraindications for co-prescriptions.[62] Certainly, those involved in prescribing drugs to patients receiving these agents need to be aware of the potential for drug interactions and those agents most commonly implicated.

References

1. Reinert RE, Hermann CG. Unexplained deaths during chlorpromazine therapy. *J Nerv Ment Dis* 1960; **131**: 435–442.
2. Kelly HQ, Fay JE, Laverty FG. Thioridazine hydrochloride (Mellaril): Its effect on the electrocardiogram and a report on two fatalities with electrographic abnormalities. *Can Med Assoc J* 1963; **89**: 546–554.
3. Desautels S, Filteau C, St Jean A. Ventricular tachycardia associated with administration of thioridazine hydrochloride (Mellaril). *Can Med Assoc J* 1964; **90**: 1030–1031.
4. Ban TA, St-Jean A. Electrocardiographic changes induced by phenothiazine drugs. *Am Heart J* 1965; **70**: 575–6.
5. Hollander PB, Cain RM. Effects of thioridazine on transmembrane potential and contractile characteristics of guinea pig hearts. *Eur J Pharmacol* 1971; **16**: 129–135.
6. Sims A, Prior P. Arteriosclerosis-related deaths in severe neurosis. *Compr Psychiatry* 1982; **23**: 181–185.
7. Baxter, DN. The mortality experience of individuals on the Salford psychiatric case register. I. All cause mortality. *Br J Psychiatry* 1996; **168**: 772–779.
8. Hansen V, Arnesen E, Jacobsen BK. Total mortality in people admitted to a psychiatric hospital. *Br J Psychiatry* 1997; **170**: 186–190.
9. Harris EC, Barraclough B. Excess mortality of mental disorder. *Br J Psychiatry* 1998; **173**: 11–53.
10. Ruschena D, Mullen PE, Burgess P, *et al*. Sudden death in psychiatric patients. *Br J Psychiatry* 1998; **172**: 331–336.
11. Schoeten EG, Dekker JM, Meppelink P, *et al*. QT interval prolongation predicts cardiovascular mortality in an apparently healthy population. *Circulation* 1991; **84**: 1516–1523.
12. Goldberg RJ, Bengtson J, Chen Z, *et al*. Duration of the QT interval and total cardiovascular mortality in healthy persons (The Framingham Study Experience). *Am J Cardiol* 1991; **67**: 55–58.
13. Moss AJ, Schwartz PJ, Crampton RS, *et al*. The long QT syndrome. Prospective

longitudinal study of 328 families. *Circulation* 1991; **84**: 1136–1144.

14. Thomas SHL. Drugs, QT interval abnormalities and ventricular arrhythmias. *Adverse Drug React Toxicol Rev* 1994; **13**: 77–102.

15. Denes P, Gabster A, Huang SK. Clinical, electrocardiographic and follow-up observations in patients having ventricular fibrillation during holter monitoring. Role of quinidine therapy. *Am J Cardiol* 1981; **48**: 9–16.

16. Bauman JL, Bauernfeind RA, Hoff JV, *et al*. *Torsades de pointes* due to quinidine: observations in 31 patients. *Am Heart J* 1984; **107**: 425–30.

17. Day CP, James OFW, Butler TJ, *et al*. QT prolongation and sudden death in patients with alcoholic liver disease. *Lancet* 1993; **341**: 1423–1428.

18. Drake WM, Broadhurst PA. QT-interval prolongation with Ecstasy. *S Afr Med J* 1996; **86**: 180–181.

19. Perera R, Kraebber A, Schwartz M. Prolonged QT interval and cocaine use. *J Electrocardiol* 1997; **30**: 337–339.

20. Merri M, Benhorin J, Alberti M, *et al*. Electrocardiographic quantitation of ventricular repolarization. *Circulation* 1989; **80**: 1301–1308

21. Rautaharju P, Zhou SH, Wong S, *et al*. Sex differences in the evolution of the electrocardiographic QT interval with age. *Can J Cardiol* 1992: **8**: 690–695.

22. Makkar RR, Fromm BS, Steinman RT, *et al*. Female gender as a risk factor for *torsades de pointes* associated with cardiovascular drugs. *JAMA* 1993; **270**: 2590–2597.

23. Drici MD, Burklow TR, Haridasse V, *et al*. Sex hormones prolong the QT interval and downregulate potassium channel expression in the rabbit heart. *Circulation* 1996; **94**: 1471–1474.

24. Stratmann HG, Kennedy HL. *Torsades de pointes* associated with drugs and toxins: Recognition and management. *Am Heart J* 1987; **113**: 1470–1482.

25. Hartigan-Go K, Bateman DN, Daly AK, *et al*. Stereoselective cardiotoxic effects of terodiline. *Clin Pharmacol Ther* 1996; **60**: 89–98.

26. Shah RR. The significance of the QT interval in drug development. *Brit J Clin Pharmacol* 2002; **54**: 188–202.

27. Mattioni TA, Zheutlin TA, Sarmiento JJ, *et al*. Amiodarone in patients with previous drug-mediated *torsades de pointes*: Long term safety and efficacy. *Ann Intern Med* 1989; **111**: 574–580.

28. Hii JTY, Wyse DG, Gillis AM, *et al*. Precordial QT interval dispersion as a marker of *torsades de pointes*: Disparate effects of class Ia antiarrhythmic drugs and amiodarone. *Circulation* 1992; **86**: 1376–1382.

29. Eckardt L, Breithardt G, Haverkamp W. Electrophysiologic characterization of the antipsychotic drug sertindole in a rabbit heart model of *torsades de pointes*: Low torsadogenic potential despite QT prolongation. *J Pharmacol Exp Ther* 2002; **300**: 64–71.

30. Fish FA, Roden DM. A prolonged QTc interval. Is it an important effect of antidysrhythmic drugs? *Med Tox Adverse Exp* 1989; **4**: 400–401.

31. Selzer A, Wray HW. Quinidine syncope: Paroxysmal ventricular fibrillation occurring during treatment of chronic atrial arrhythmias. *Circulation* 1964; **31**: 17–26.

32. Roden DM, Woosley RL, Primm RK. Incidence and clinical features of the quinidine-associated long QT syndrome: Implications for patient care. *Am Heart J* 1986; **111**: 1088–1093.

33. Warner JP, Barnes TRE, Henry JA. Electrocardiographic changes in patients receiving neuroleptic medication. *Acta Psychiatr Scand* 1996; **93**: 311–313.

34. Reilly JG, Ayis SA, Ferrier IN, *et al*. QT interval abnormalities and psychotropic drug therapy in psychiatric patients. *Lancet* 2000; **355**: 1048–1052.

35. Ray WA, Meredith S, Thapa PB, *et al*. Antipsychotics and the risk of sudden cardiac death. *Arch Gen Psychiatr* 2001; **58**: 1161–1167.

36. Thomas SHL, Higham PD, Hartigan-Go K, *et al*. Concentration related cardiotoxic effects of terodiline in patients treated for urinary incontinence. *Br Heart J* 1995; **74**: 53–56.

37. Dancey D, Wulffhart Z, McEwan P. Sotalol-induced *torsades de pointes* in patients with renal failure. *Canadian Journal of Cardiology* 1997; **13**: 55–58.

38. Okumura K, Kita T, Chikazawa S, Komada F, Iwakawa S, Tanigawara Y. Genotyping of N-acetylation polymorphism and correlation with procainamide metabolism. *Clinical Pharmacology & Therapeutics* 1997; **61**: 509–517.

39. Woosley RL. Antiarrhythmic drugs. *Annu Rev Pharmacol Toxicol* 1991; **31**: 427–55.

40. Von Bahr C, Movin G, Nordin C, *et al*. Plasma concentrations of thioridazine and metabolites are influenced by the debrisoquin hydroxylation phenotype. *Clin*

Pharmacol Ther 1991; **49**: 234–40.

41. Hartigan-Go K, Bateman DN, Nyberg G, *et al*. Concentration-related pharmacodynamic effects of thioridazine and its metabolites in humans. *Clin Pharmacol Ther* 1996; **60**: 543–553.

42. Connolly MJ, Astridge PS, White EG, *et al*. *Torsades de pointes* ventricular tachycardia and terodiline. *Lancet* 1991; **338**: 344–345.

43. McCloud AA, Thorogood S, Barnett S. *Torsades de pointes* complicating treatment with terodiline. *BMJ* 1991; **302**: 1469.

44. Hippisley-Cox J, Pringle M, Hammersley V, *et al*. Antidepressants as a risk factor for ischaemic heart disease: Case-control study in primary care. *Brit Med J* 2001; **323**: 666–669.

45. Monahan BP, Ferguson CL, Killeavy ES, *et al*. Torsades de points occurring in association with terfenadine use. *JAMA* 1990; **264**: 2788–2790.

46. Woosley RL, Chen Y, Freiman JP, *et al*. Mechanism of the cardiotoxic actions of terfenadine. *JAMA* 1993; **269**: 1532–6.

47. Cisapride (Prepulsid): Risk of arrhythmias. Committee on Safety of Medicines. *Current problems in pharmacovigilance* 1998; **24**: 1–2.

48. Flockhart DA, Drici MD, Kerbusch T, *et al*. Studies on the mechanism of a fatal clarithromycin-pimozide interaction in a patient with Tourette syndrome. *J Clin Psychopharmacol* 2000; **20**: 317–24.

49. Jusic N, Lader M. Post-mortem antipsychotic drug concentrations and unexplained deaths. *Br J Psychiatry* 1994; **165**: 787–791.

50. Lereya J, Segal A, Elizur A. Sudden death, neuroleptics and psychotic agitation. *Prog Neuropsychopharmacol Biol Psychiatry* 1995; **19**: 229–241.

51. Reilly JG, Ayis SA, Ferrier IN, *et al*. Thioridazine and sudden unexplained death in psychiatric in-patients. *Brit J Psychiatry* 2002; **180**: 515–522.

52. Mehtonen OP, Aranko K, Malkonen L, *et al*. A survey of sudden death associated with the use of antipsychotic or antidepressant drugs: 49 cases in Finland. *Acta Psychiat Scand* 1991; **84**: 58–64.

53. Suspension of the availability of sertindole. Committee on Safety of Medicines. *Current problems in pharmacovigilance* 1999; **25**: 1.

54. Glassman AH, Bigger JT. Antipsychotic drugs: prolonged QTc interval, *torsades de pointes*, and sudden death. *American Journal of Psychiatry* 2001; **158**: 1774–1782.

55. Drolet B, Vincent F, Rail J, *et al*. Thioridazine lengthens repolarization of cardiac ventricular myocytes by blocking the delayed rectifier potassium current. *J Pharmacol Exp Ther* 1999; **288**: 1261–8.

56. Buckley NA, Whyte IM, Dawson AH. Cardiotoxicity more common in thioridazine overdose than other neuroleptics. *J Toxicol Clin Toxicol* 1995; **33**: 199–204.

57. Appleby L, Thomas S, Ferrier N, *et al*. Sudden unexplained death in psychiatric in-patients. *Br J Psychiatry* 2000; **176**: 405–406.

58. Albert CM, Manson JE, Cook NR, *et al*. Moderate alcohol consumption and the risk of sudden cardiac death among US male physicians. *Circulation* 1999; **100**: 944–950.

59. Jouven X, Desnoos NM, Guerot C, *et al*. Predicting sudden death in the population: The Paris prospective Study I. *Circulation* 1999; **99**: 1978–1983.

60. Koro CE, Fedder DO, L'Italien GJ, *et al*. Assessment of independent effect of olanzapine and risperidone on risk of diabetes among patients with schizophrenia: Population-based nested case-control study. *BMJ* 2002; **325**: 243–5.

61. The Maudsley 2001 Prescribing Guidelines. Taylor D, McConnell H, McConnell D, *et al*. (ed). London: Martin Dunitz Ltd, 2001; pp14.

62. Yap YG, Camm J. Risk of *torsades de pointes* with non-cardiac drugs. *BMJ* 2000; **320**: 1158–1159.

63. Dahl M-L, Bertilsson L. Genetically variable metabolism of antidepressants and neuroleptic drugs in man. *Pharmacogenetics* 1993; **3**: 61–70.

64. Goldberg RJ. The P-450 system: Definition and relevance to the use of antidepressants in medical practice. *Arch Fam Med* 1996; **5**: 406–412.

65. Nemeroff CB, DeVane CL, Pollock BG. Newer antidepressants and the cytochrome P450 system. *Am J Psychiatry* 1996; **153**: 311–20.

66. Elliott R. Pharmacokinetic drug interactions of newer antidepressants: A review of the effects on the metabolism of other drugs. *Mayo Clin Proc* 1997; **72**: 835–847.

67. Bertilsson L, Dahl M-L, Dalen P, *et al*. Molecular genetics of CYP2D6: Clinical relevance with focus on psychotropic drugs. *Brit J Clin Pharmacol* 2002; **53**: 111–122.

QT interval prolongation in perspective

A. John Camm,

Professor of Clinical Cardiology, Department of Cardiological Sciences,
St. George's Hospital and Medical School, London, United Kingdom.

Correspondence: Professor A. John Camm, MD, FRCP,

Professor of Clinical Cardiology,

Department of Cardiological Sciences,

St. George's Hospital Medical School, Cranmer Terrace,

London, SW17 0RE.

Telephone: +44 (0)20 8725 3554

Facsimile: +44 (0)20 8767 7141

Email: jcamm@sghms.ac.uk

1. Risk of schizophrenia and antipsychotic therapy

Mortality in people with schizophrenia is substantially higher (about double) than in the general population. The increased mortality is due to natural and unnatural causes (e.g. suicide). A large component of the increased mortality in this population is undoubtedly due to cardiovascular disease. Although some of the increased risk of cardiovascular disease is due to limited access to and use of medical care and poor insight into medial status, a significant proportion is related to increased prevalence of risk factors, such as smoking, reduced activity, diabetes, hypertension, and hyperlipidemia. People with schizophrenia also have a high incidence of metabolic syndrome which is, in part, related to the antipsychotic therapy that they receive.

The combination of three or more of the following: obesity (e.g. increased girth measurements and weight), hypercholesterolemia, hypertriglyceridemia, glucose intolerance (often with raised blood glucose), and hypertension constitutes metabolic syndrome. This constellation of factors, which presents an enormous cardiovascular risk, is increasingly common (up to 25% of the adult population of the USA) and has been associated with some antipsychotic agents but not others. Obesity, hyperlipidemia and glucose intolerance have particularly been noted in association with both typical and atypical antipsychotics.

The most common basis for sudden death in schizophrenia is coronary heart disease, but ventricular arrhythmia due to prolongation of the QT interval induced by antipsychotic drugs has been proposed as a significant cause. Some typical antipsychotics, such as thioridazine and pimozide, have a marked effect on the QT interval and *torsades de pointes* has been documented in association with their use. However, some atypical antipsychotics also prolong the QT interval and the occasional episode of *torsades de pointes* has been documented in patients receiving some of these therapies. The issue of QT prolongation has loomed very large and very far out of proportion with respect to these new therapies.

2. QT interval as a risk factor

In the general population the duration of the QT interval has sometimes been shown to be associated with an increased risk of mortality.[1-4] However, other studies have not confirmed this relationship.[5-6] Similarly, in patients after myocardial infarction or with congestive heart failure QT prolongation has been variously shown to confer risk, or to be harmless.[7-11] There are few studies in patients with schizophrenia, but there is a suggestion that increased QT interval is associated with increased risk of mortality.[12-13] However, the risk of QT prolongation is minor compared with the conventional risk factors for coronary artery disease.

Since antipsychotic therapy may prolong the QT interval it has been suggested that an ECG should be taken in all patients prior to antipsychotic therapy with agents known to prolong the QT interval. This may be useful in order to uncover unsuspected underlying heart disease, and the rare case of inherited or acquired long QT syndrome. Similarly an on-treatment ECG might provide useful information about the effect of a therapy on the duration of ventricular repolarisation for particular patients. However, ECG recording is not a simple procedure, the ECG may be difficult to interpret, and the test is expensive to perform routinely.

3. ECG recordings prior to therapy

There is no doubt that the patient's medical history should be ascertained prior to the prescription of any of the current antipsychotic agents. Of relevance to treatment with antipsychotic agents, the history should reveal prior cardiac disease and past episodes of syncope or arrhythmia. Similarly, a family history of syncope, sudden death or inherited cardiac conditions should also emerge. The patient or his/her relatives/carers should also be able to supply information about concomitant therapy with other drugs that prolong the QT interval (e.g. class Ia and class III antiarrhythmic agents) or promote hypokalaemia (such as potassium wasting diuretics). A reasonable medical history should allow most patients at potential risk from antipsychotic therapy to be further investigated (including ECG where appropriate), with a view to a full assessment of their risk of QT prolongation and their suitability for therapy with these agents.

Routine ECG prior to prescription of therapy would seem to be a wise precaution. However, the technique is neither sensitive nor specific for distinguishing symptomatic or asymptomatic gene-positive long QT syndrome subjects from their relatives without the gene.[14] ECGs are very highly variable even in members of the same family with the same gene defect.[15] The ECG is particularly unhelpful in children. For example, it has been calculated that recording an ECG in 1000,000 children and using a QTc cut off of 500 ms would identify 61 of 200 affected children, and 100 unaffected children.[16] Automatic ECG recordings aggravate the situation further. Miller and colleagues,[17] showed that computer generated ECG diagnostic interpretation erroneously classified six of 23 family members and, further, that "half of the family members, proved to have the ion channel defect, received the diagnostic interpretation "normal ECG."

It is widely understood that the long QT syndromes vary considerably with respect to genetic penetrance of their ECG-related phenotype. It is also generally well known that only a small percentage of drug-induced long QT syndromes are related to the monogenic disorders that are responsible for congenital long QT syndromes. Thus, although approximately 80% of the congenital long QT syndromes have been genotyped, very few (approximately 11%),[18] of the acquired long QT syndromes are associated with an underlying functionally important genetic variant. About another 10 – 15% may be due in part to polymorphisms in pore-forming genes which would not, however, cause any abnormality of the baseline ECG.

In summary, a baseline ECG would be valuable in patients with a past medical history or family history suggestive of a long QT channelopathy, and in patients with significant cardiac disease. Screening electrocardiography in order to detect underlying vulnerability to risk from QT prolonging drugs is otherwise inefficient, costly and potentially misleading.

4. ECG recordings during therapy
4.1 Powerful QT-prolonging drugs (*torsades de pointes* in 1 to 5 per 10^2 of exposed patients)

It is undoubtedly correct that in most subjects the QT interval (or QTc) is markedly prolonged (usually beyond 500 ms) at or about the time that the patient experiences *torsades de pointes* due to the administration of a QT-prolonging drug.[19] Drugs that exert powerful blockade of I_{Kr} (or other relevant membrane channel), such as class III antiarrhythmic agents, may cause an immediate and marked QT prolongation that can be detected on ECG recordings within a few days of starting therapy. Indeed, with such drugs, the majority of instances of *torsades de pointes* also occur early in the course of therapy.[20–21] Such a marked QT response, which can be detected by continuous ECG monitoring during the first several days of therapy, should be used to prompt a decrease in the drug dose, or suspension of therapy with that agent. There are probably no antipsychotic drugs in this category.

4.2 Intermediate QT-prolonging drugs (*torsades de pointes* in 1 per 10^3 – 10^4 of exposed patients)

Drugs that notably prolong the QT interval at ordinary dosages may induce massive QT prolongation when taken in large overdose, or when the metabolism or excretion of the drug is compromised. Terfenadine and cisapride are the classical examples of this situation. Inhibition of the cytochrome CYP3A4 leads to accumulation of the parent drug and gross QT prolongation, leading to *torsades de pointes* in a small proportion of patients. Sertindole is an antipsychotic which has this potential risk.

Chlorpromazine, thioridazine and pimozide induce prominent QT prolongation at ordinary dosages, and have been reported to be associated not infrequently with *torsades de pointes* and/or sudden death; overdose with such agents poses a particular risk.

Under these circumstances, it is generally recommended that an ECG is recorded routinely prior to, and following, initiation of treatment. The ECG prior to treatment serves as a baseline, and may also reveal unsuspected cardiac disease and QT prolongation. After therapy has started, an on-therapy ECG may reveal undue prolongation of the of QT interval (QTc >500 ms). In this situation, therapy should be discontinued unless absolutely necessary. If therapy is continued regular ECG and electrolyte monitoring should be undertaken.

4.3 Drugs that induce mild-to-moderate QT prolongation (*torsades de pointes* in 1 per $10^5 - 10^7$ exposed patients)

Some drugs that prolong the QT interval by only a few milliseconds in the usual state may induce more marked and potentially serious prolongation when other co-factors are present. Slight prolongation is masked by a host of variables that confound accurate assessment of small QT changes:

- inaccuracy and inconsistency of manual measurement of the QT interval (high inter- and intra-observer errors)
- lack of relationship between computer-derived and manual measurement of the QT interval,[22] although computer derived QT measurements are more reproducible[23]
- uncertainty relating to the methods of correcting the QT interval for the ambient heart rate environment and the immediately preceding RR intervals[24] – individual corrections are probably needed to be sufficiently accurate to tease out significant QT interval changes[25]
- diurnal QT variability of up to 95 ms.[26]

Thus, the major finding in any data set that compares a baseline ECG with an ECG recorded after treatment with a drug that causes mild-to-moderate QT prolongation is characterised by "regression to the mean". Thus, those with longer baseline QT values tend to have shorter on treatment values, and vice versa. Such was the case when this type of analysis was performed on the patients treated with ziprasidone.

If *torsades de pointes* is to occur with drugs of this nature other co-factors must be present. These include:

- bradycardia and long pauses, which occur in fit young people as well as older patients with sinus node disease. Several groups of drugs, such as beta-blockers or calcium antagonists, induce or aggravate this problem
- hypokalemia and hypomagnesaemia (which may occur in patients taking potassium wasting diuretics or suffering from vomiting and diarrhoea
- co-administration of another QT prolonging therapy, including other antipsychotics and tricyclic antidepressants, etc.

None of these co-factors is better predicted by an on-therapy ECG than by the medical history and physical examination of the patient.

The added value of an on-treatment ECG in such circumstances is an assessment of T wave distortion. However, this type of evaluation is difficult even for experts to describe or repeat accurately. The automatic ECG machine QT interval algorithms also perform inconsistently when the T wave is flat or distorted.[27]

Therefore, a routine on-treatment ECG is not sufficiently sensitive, accurate or practical to be recommended for patients taking drugs such as quetiapine, risperidone, haloperidol, or ziprasidone, which are not expected to result in gross QT prolongation, or lead to *torsades de pointes* in more than a very rare instance.

Most typical and several atypical antipsychotic drugs prolong the QT interval, but it is now well understood that, in itself, drug-induced QT prolongation does not necessarily imply that ventricular arrhythmias will ensue. Present experience suggests that *torsades de pointes* is no more than a rare complication which ought to be very largely eliminated by taking a good medical, drug and family history. The risk with antipsychotic agents should be several orders of magnitude less than with class III antiarrhythmic agents (degree of I_{Kr} blocking effect), and much less than terfenadine or cisapride (little or no metabolic/elimination jeopardy).

The typical antipsychotics, thioridazine, pimozide and chlorpromazine, may be complicated more often than others by marked QT prolongation and *torsades de pointes*, and routine ECG is advised to reduce the risk of these unwanted and serious complications. However, for treatment with the majority of antipsychotics, a routine on-treatment ECG will not entirely abolish risk, but may give potentially misleading results, and present a practical and expensive barrier to their use.

5. Global assessment of risk

Cardiovascular disease (coronary artery disease) is the single, leading cause of death in Western societies, and is becoming increasingly more relevant in developing countries. People with schizophrenia have far greater risk of developing this potentially fatal disease than the general adult population. The choice of antipsychotic therapy may add to this risk by increasing major risk factors for coronary artery disease. Therapy might also expose the patients to some small risk from prolongation of ventricular repolarisation. In conclusion, the risk of QT prolongation and consequent ventricular arrhythmia is relatively insignificant compared with the considerable risk from coronary artery disease.

References

1. Schouten EG, Dekker JM, Meppelink P, et al. QT interval prolongation predicts cardiovascular mortality in an apparently healthy population. Circulation 1991; **84**: 1516–1523.

2. Elming H, Holm E, Jun L, et al. The prognostic value of the QT interval and QT interval dispersion in all-cause and cardiac mortality and morbidity in a population of Danish citizens. Eur Heart J 1998; **19**: 1391–400.

3. de Bruyne MC, Hoes AW, Kors JA, et al. Prolonged QT interval predicts cardiac and all-cause mortality in the elderly. The Rotterdam Study. Eur Heart J 1999; **20**: 278–84.

4. Okin PM, Devereux RB, Howard BV, et al. Assessment of QT interval and QT dispersion for prediction of all-cause and cardiovascular mortality in American Indians: The Strong Heart Study. Circulation 2000; **101**: 61–6.

5. Ahnve S. Is QT interval prolongation a strong or weak predictor for cardiac death? Circulation 1991; **84**: 1862–1865.

6. Goldberg RJ, Bengtson J, Chen ZY, et al. Duration of the QT interval and total and cardiovascular mortality in healthy persons (The Framingham Heart Study experience). Am J Cardiol 1991; **67**: 55–58.

7. Schwartz PJ, Wolf S. QT interval prolongation as predictor of sudden death in patients with myocardial infarction. Circulation 1978; **57**: 1074–1077.

8. Wheelan K, Mukharji J, Rude RE, et al. Sudden death and its relation to QT-interval prolongation after acute myocardial infarction: Two-year follow-up. Am J Cardiol 1986; **57**: 745–750.

9. Dekker JM, Schouten EG, Klootwijk P, et al. Association between QT interval and coronary heart disease in middle-aged and elderly men. The Zutphen Study. Circulation 1994; **90**: 779–785.

10. Tobe TJ, de Langen CD, Crijns HJ, et al. Late potentials, QTc prolongation, and prediction of arrhythmic events after myocardial infarction. Int J Cardiol 1994; **46**: 121–128.

11. Brooksby P, Batin PD, Nolan J, et al. The relationship between QT intervals and mortality in ambulant patients with chronic heart failure. The united kingdom heart failure evaluation and assessment of